FIFTH EDITION

Nutrition AND Dietetics

Practice and Future Trends

Esther A. Winterfeldt, PhD

Professor Emeritus, Department of Nutritional Sciences
College of Human Environmental Sciences
Oklahoma State University
Stillwater, Oklahoma

Margaret L. Bogle, PhD

Retired
Active Member of the Academy of Nutrition and Dietetics
Dallas, Texas

Lea L. Ebro, PhD

Professor Emeritus, Department of Nutritional Sciences
College of Human Environmental Sciences
Oklahoma State University
Stillwater, Oklahoma

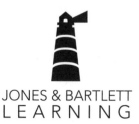

JONES & BARTLETT
LEARNING

World Headquarters
Jones & Bartlett Learning
5 Wall Street
Burlington, MA 01803
978-443-5000
info@jblearning.com
www.jblearning.com

Production Credits

VP, Executive Publisher: David D. Cella
Publisher: Cathy L. Esperti
Acquisitions Editor: Sean Fabery
Associate Editor: Taylor Maurice
Production Assistant: Molly Hogue
Director of Marketing: Andrea DeFronzo
VP, Manufacturing and Inventory Control: Therese Connell

Composition: Cenveo® Publisher Services
Cover Design: Theresa Manley
Rights & Media Specialist: Merideth Tumasz
Media Development Editor: Shannon Sheehan
Cover Image: © Bounce/Getty Images
Printing and Binding: Edwards Brothers Malloy
Cover Printing: Edwards Brothers Malloy

Library of Congress Cataloging-in-Publication Data

Names: Winterfeldt, Esther A., author. | Bogle, Margaret L., author. | Ebro, Lea L., author.
Title: Nutrition and dietetics : practice and future trends / Esther A. Winterfeldt, PhD, Professor Emeritus, Department of Nutritional Sciences, College of Human Environmental Sciences, Oklahoma State University, Stillwater, Oklahoma, Margaret L. Bogle, PhD, RD, LD, Lower Mississippi Delta Nutrition Intervention Research Initiative, Agriculture Research Service, United States Department of Agriculture, Little Rock, Arkansas, Lea L. Ebro, PhD, Professor Emeritus, Department of Nutritional Sciences, College of Human Environmental Sciences, Oklahoma State University, Stillwater, Oklahoma.
Other titles: Dietetics (Winterfeldt)
Description: Fifth edition. | Burlington, MA : Jones & Bartlett Learning, [2018] | Revision of: Dietetics / Esther A. Winterfeldt, Margaret L. Bogle, Lea L. Ebro. 3rd ed. c2011. | Includes bibliographical references and index.
Identifiers: LCCN 2016049226 | ISBN 9781284107975 (alk. paper)
Subjects: LCSH: Dietetics—Vocational guidance.
Classification: LCC RM217 .W56 2018 | DDC 613.2023—dc23 LC record available at https://lccn.loc.gov/2016049226

6048

Printed in the United States of America
21 20 19 18 17   10 9 8 7 6 5 4 3 2 1

Contents

Preface

As in previous editions, *Nutrition and Dietetics: Practice and Future Trends, Fifth Edition* presents an overall look at the dietetic profession—what dietitians do, where they practice, and the education and experiences needed to become a credentialed, fully prepared dietitian, nutritionist, and dietetic technician. For this edition, we have updated all the chapters, added a chapter on the government and military, and looked extensively at all references.

Our profession is focused on helping patients, clients, and the public to maintain healthy lifestyles that help prevent the onset of chronic disease and enhance the quality of life throughout the life cycle. Through educational programs, research, and many forms of communication, reliable and relevant information is provided for the public, consumers, and clients.

Dietitian nutritionists, through their unique knowledge of both the science and art of nutrition, are leaders in the promotion of nutritional health today. Because of this blend of scientific knowledge and the social and cultural factors that influence what people eat, dietitian nutritionists are able to use their skills to help individuals in illness and disease prevention as well as those who are healthy and active. Dietitian nutritionists also interact with professionals in other disciplines and are able to blend their assorted expertise for the benefit of clients. Their participation in basic research and integration of new scientific concepts into all areas of practice adds an invaluable dimension to the dietetic profession.

This text is geared toward students beginning in dietetics, those who may be undecided about a career choice, and those who are nearing completion of their education and training and exploring career opportunities. Job opportunities for the non-RD are also included throughout the text. In addition, dietitians and nutritionists considering a career change will find information about many career options, including some new emerging opportunities. Some may become entrepreneurs and join the business world, some may partner with other professionals in health care institutions to provide their expertise for clients, and some may become consultants and others may become educators and researchers. The opportunities for food and nutrition professionals are greater today than at any time in the past, and we encourage students to fully explore the many career possibilities.

Readers will find updated information regarding education, credentialing, salary data, and position descriptions. The reader will note that references are inclusive through mid-2016. The Academy will be publishing practice audit results later in 2016 and some position papers are currently under revision with an expected 2016 publication date.

We thank the Academy of Nutrition and Dietetics headquarters staff for timely information. We also acknowledge and thank other professionals who contributed to this text by sharing their knowledge and expertise in this and previous editions.

We encourage faculties and students to make full use of information sources provided as well as others which will lend further details in topic areas. We hope readers will be stimulated to participate in and enjoy the privileges of helping others through the practice of nutrition and dietetics.

New to This Edition

Each chapter has been reviewed and revised for the *Fifth Edition*. Notable changes include the following:

- Chapter 9, "Dietitians in the Government and Military Services," is new to this edition and discusses the roles of dietitians within government and military organizations as well as public policy.
- Chapter 15, "The Future in Dietetics and Nutrition," has been completely rewritten to discuss future opportunities due to changes in the field as well as future educational needs as indicated both by the Academy of Nutrition and Dietetics and employers of dietitians.
- Chapter 8, "The Public Health/Community Health Nutrition Dietitian," has been extensively revised to streamline the discussion of community and public health in relation to each other.
- Chapter 5, "The Nutrition and Dietetics Professional," discusses diversity in greater detail.

- Charts and tables throughout the text have been updated to reflect the latest salary and Academy membership data for dietitians.

Instructor Resources

Qualified instructors can receive access to the full suite of Instructor Resources for the *Fifth Edition*, including the following:

- Test Bank
- Slides in PowerPoint format
- Lecture Outlines

Esther A. Winterfeldt, PhD
Margaret L. Bogle, PhD
Lea L. Ebro, PhD

Reviewers

Susan E. Adams, MS, RD, LDN, FAND
Assistant Professor
La Salle University
Philadelphia, PA

Melissa Anderson, PhD, RD, LDN
Director, School of Human Ecology
Tennessee Tech University
Cookeville, TN

Cynthia Blanton, PhD, RD
Associate Professor
Idaho State University
Pocatello, ID

Detri Brech, PhD, RD, LD, CDE
Professor
Ouachita Baptist University
Arkadelphia, AR

Judi Brooks, PhD, RD
Professor
Eastern Michigan University
Ypsilanti, MI

Eileen Chopnick, MBA, RDN, LDN
Adjunct Faculty
La Salle University
Philadelphia, PA

Barbara Lloyd, MA, RD
Assistant Professor
Southwest Tennessee Community College
Memphis, TN

Diane Longstreet, PhD, MPH, RD, LDN
Instructor
Keiser University
Lakeland, FL

Jaimette McCulley, MS, RD, LD
Assistant Professor
Fontbonne University
St. Louis, MO

Katie Miner, PhD, RDN, LD
Senior Instructor
University of Idaho
Moscow, ID

Deborah Myers, EdD, RD
Professor
Bluffton University
Bluffton, OH

Patricia H. Terry, PhD, RD, LD
Professor and Dietetics Program Director
Samford University
Birmingham, AL

Peggy Turner, MS, RD/LD, FAND
Assistant Professor
The University of Oklahoma Health Sciences Center
Oklahoma City, OK

Kit Werner, PhD, RD, CD, CDE
Clinical Assistant Professor and Nutritional Science Clinical Director
University of Wisconsin—Milwaukee
Milwaukee, WI

CHAPTER 1

Introduction to the Profession of Nutrition and Dietetics

"An honorable past lies behind, a developing present is with us, and a promising future lies before us."[1]

OUTLINE

- Learning Objectives
- Introduction
- The Early Practice of Dietetics
  - Cooking Schools
  - Hospital Dietetics
  - Clinics
  - The Military
- Founding of the Academy of Nutrition and Dietetics
- Influential Leaders
  - Recognized Leaders Today
- Dietetics as a Profession
- Growth of the Profession
  - Membership
  - Registration and Licensure
  - The Academy of Nutrition and Dietetics Foundation
  - Dietetic Technicians and Managers
  - Legislative Activity
  - Areas of Practice

- · Dietetic Practice Groups
- · Long-Range Planning
- · Professional Partnerships
- · Reaching Out to the Public
- · Historical Events in the Academy of Nutrition and Dietetics
- · Summary
- · Definitions
- · References

LEARNING OBJECTIVES

The student will be able to:

1. Describe early practices in dietetics.
2. Become familiar with the founding of the Academy of Nutrition and Dietetics.
3. Discuss how the profession has grown since inception.
4. Become familiar with names of early leaders in the profession and their contributions.
5. Name and describe the primary practice areas in dietetics.

INTRODUCTION

"What is a dietitian?" "What does a dietitian do?"

Recognition of the dietitian as a food and nutrition expert became official in 1917. This, however, was not the actual beginning of the practice of dietetics. The use of diet in the treatment of disease was already an ancient practice even though it was based more on trial and error than on scientific knowledge. Besides physicians, others including home economists, nurses, and cooks were practicing and teaching about good dietary practices, and researchers were uncovering the secrets of nutrients in foods and their health-promoting effect.[2]

Dietetics has been practiced as long as people have been eating. The term derives from *dieto*, meaning diet or food. According to earliest historical evidence, our ancestors were forced to concentrate on simply finding food with little concern about the variety or composition of that food. Today, however, food is plentiful. At least in the developed countries of the world, being able to choose and eat too much from that abundant food supply has become a major problem, resulting in adverse health for many.

Recommendations about eating and food choices have come from biblical admonitions as well as from early physicians and scientists. Physicians in Europe and China, including Hippocrates, formed theories about the relationship between food and the state of a person's health.[3] Many of the early physicians and scientists emphasized adding or eliminating certain foods from the diet according to disease symptoms, although there was no knowledge at that time about nutrients. Until the discovery of the major nutrients in food during the 19th and 20th centuries, a scientific basis for many of the eating recommendations was tenuous at best.

During the 18th century, research by chemists and physicians began to yield information concerning digestion, respiration, and other metabolic functions. The studies were forerunners of later discoveries that identified the elusive substances in foods that were responsible for many of the effects described much earlier in the etiology of disease. Fats, carbohydrates, and amines were known by the mid-1800s, but vitamins and minerals were not discovered until the early 1900s.[4]

One of the most fascinating accounts of the relationship between specific foods and illness is found in Lind's *Treatise of Scurvy* written in 1753.[5] When it was discovered that lemons and limes or their juice would prevent the dreaded scurvy among sailors at sea for long periods of time, it was a lifesaving piece of knowledge. Vitamin C from citrus fruits was later termed the *antiscorbutic* vitamin. Other breakthroughs came when vitamin A was found to be a factor in the prevention of skin lesions and blindness in both animals and people, and when niacin, one of the B-vitamin group, was found to prevent pellagra in humans and black tongue in dogs.[6] There are equally vivid accounts of discoveries of other nutrients.[7]

THE EARLY PRACTICE OF DIETETICS

Cooking Schools

Early cooking schools in the United States, following their emergence in Europe in the early 1800s, led the way toward good dietary practices.[8] One of the first was the New York Cooking Academy founded in 1876, soon followed by schools in Boston and Philadelphia.[9] The schools not only offered cooking instruction but conducted laboratories in chemistry and special classes for the sick.[10] The schools trained many of the men and women who were in charge of food service in hospitals and the Red Cross during World War I.

Hospital Dietetics

Early practitioners in dietetics were in hospitals feeding the sick. Because little was known about people's nutritional needs in either health or illness, food selection was not a major concern. Menus were monotonous and usually featured only a few foods. One account of menus in a New York hospital indicated that mush, molasses, and beer were served for breakfast and supper several days a week. Fruits and vegetables did not appear on menus until later, and then usually only as a garnish.[11]

Florence Nightingale is credited not only with improving nursing of the sick during the Crimean War in the mid-1800s but also with improving the food supply and sanitary conditions in hospitals.[12]

Clinics

The Frances Stern Clinic in Boston was one of the leading food clinics established in the late 1800s to provide diets for the sick poor. This clinic continues as a leading treatment center and serves as a model for similar clinics throughout the United States.

The Military

Dietitians played important roles during the Civil War and World Wars I and II. During World War I, many served in military hospitals both overseas and in the United States. In World War II during the 1940s, hundreds of dietitians volunteered for active service. Dietitians also worked closely with the Office of the Surgeon General and the Red Cross to help train more individuals in nutrition. Military service and training programs are important professional opportunities for dietitians today.[13]

FOUNDING OF THE ACADEMY OF NUTRITION AND DIETETICS

The history of the profession of dietetics in the United Stated is also the history of the American Dietetic Association (ADA; now called the Academy of Nutrition and Dietetics) because the two grew together in increasingly important ways. The profession flourished because the association took early steps to oversee both the education and practice of its members. In turn, dietitians supported the association and its activities.

Before the founding of the ADA, persons who worked in food and nutrition programs could join the American Home Economics Association and thus were able to associate and communicate with others of like interests. Dietitians were few in number, and, although they had somewhat similar backgrounds, there was no way to identify persons who were professionally qualified. In 1917, a group of about 100 dietitians met in Cleveland, Ohio, for the purpose of "providing an opportunity for the dietitians of the country to come together and meet with the scientific research workers and to see that the feeding of as many people as possible be placed in the hands of women trained to feed them in the best manner known."[14] Because this was wartime, the government had extensive food conservation programs and used home economists, dietitians, and volunteers to conduct the programs. At the first meeting of the association, officers were elected and a constitution and bylaws were drawn up overnight. Dues were $1 per year, and there were 39 charter members. Lulu Grace Graves was the first president, and Lenna Frances Cooper was the first vice president.

World War I was, in great part, the impetus that brought early dietitians together to discuss the feeding needs. However, it was also recognized that the services of dietitians in hospitals were rapidly assuming greater importance, both in food service and in treating illness with diet. Researchers were making great strides in nutrition science, and, as more became known about nutrients, maintaining good nutrition and treating certain illnesses with diet became more precise.

Four areas of practice in dietetics were first identified: dietotherapy, teaching, social welfare, and administration.[15] The vision of the early leaders is evident in that the same four areas of practice exist today, although terminology as well as practice in each area have undergone many changes. The first area, dietotherapy, or the treatment of disease by diet, was later termed *diet therapy*, then *clinical dietetics*, and now is known as *medical nutrition therapy* or *clinical nutrition*. Dietitians instructed dietetics students, nurses, physicians, and patients. Later called the *education section*, this group established education standards and specified the experiences needed in an internship to become professionally competent. The social welfare area of practice was later named *community nutrition*. The administration practice became known as institution administration and later food systems management or management in food and nutrition.

The association continued to grow and by 1927 had 1200 members. The office headquarters were located in Chicago, and the association was legally incorporated in the state of Illinois. The first edition of the *Journal of the American Dietetic Association* was published in 1925, with four issues per year. Early issues of the journal featured subjects similar to those published today, such as hospital food service, personnel issues, and special diets, especially the diabetic diet.

INFLUENTIAL LEADERS

Sarah Tyson Rorer has been credited as the first American dietitian. She was an instructor in one of the early cooking schools and educated both dietitians and physicians in hospital dietetics. Ellen H. Richards was the founder and leader of the home economics movement and so is claimed as one of the early leaders in dietetics. Lulu Graves served as the first president of the ADA and established a training course for hospital dietitians at Cornell University. Lenna Frances Cooper was an early ADA president and director of the School of Home Economics at Battle Creek Health Care Institution in Michigan. Later, she was appointed to the staff of the U.S. surgeon general in Washington, DC. She is commemorated through a lecture presented each year at the annual meeting of the ADA by a current leader in the profession.[16]

Ruth Wheeler prepared the first outline of a training course for student dietitians that established education requirements for dietetics practice. Mary E. Barber, another ADA president, was the director of home economics at Battle Creek and was appointed as a food consultant in 1941 to assist with the problems of feeding 1.5 million soldiers in World War II. She also edited the first official history of the ADA. Mary Swartz Rose was a leader in nutrition research and nutrition education for the public and established the Department of Nutrition at Columbia University. The Mary Swartz Rose fellowship for graduate study is awarded yearly in honor of this outstanding scientist and scholar.[17]

Mary P. Huddleston was the editor of the ADA journal from 1927 to 1946. An annual award is presented in her name to the author of the best article published in the previous year's journal. Anna Boller Beach was the first executive secretary of the ADA in 1923, served as president, and was the historian of the association for many years. Lydia J. Roberts was a leading nutritionist at the University of Chicago and the University of Puerto Rico. She initiated nutrition education programs to improve the nutritional status of children in Puerto Rico and was recognized widely for this accomplishment. Mary deGarmo Bryan inspected hospital training courses for dietitians in the 1930s and also developed a training course for directors of school lunch programs.

Scores of other influential leaders led the way in dietetics. Additional information can be found in *Carry the Flame: The History of the American Dietetic Association*[18] and in several issues of the Academy journal. This brief listing highlights those leaders who played key roles in founding the association and thus were pioneers in the profession of dietetics.

Many influential leaders have stepped forth over the years to assume leadership positions that moved the Association forward. The historical series of articles beginning in 2012 (shown later in this chapter) point to many persons and events important in the growing profession. A 2013 President's page made reference to several leaders in specific areas of practice.[19]

Recognized Leaders Today

Each year, the Academy selects leaders who have made significant contributions to the profession and are singled out for recognition at the annual meeting. The highest honor awarded is the Marjorie Hulsizer Copher Award for which one recipient is named each year. The award is given in recognition of Copher who had a distinguished career in WWI, having been decorated by both England and France for improving food service delivery in field hospitals before serving as chief dietitian at Barnes Hospital in St. Louis. The awardee is a leader who has shown extensive, active participation and service to the profession of dietetics nutrition. The complete listing of persons receiving the honor can be accessed on the Academy website.

The Medallion Awards are presented each year to several (5 to 10) Academy members who have demonstrated outstanding service to the profession in various ways. Dietitian nutritionists who have been members of the Academy for at least 10 years are eligible to be nominated. All past recipients are also listed on the Academy website.

Another honor awarded each year is for a member selected to present the Lenna Frances Cooper Memorial Lecture. The person receiving the award presents a lecture on a topic of his/her choice at the annual meeting, which is published later in the journal. Persons selected are accomplished speakers as well as having made unique contributions to the profession.

In 2015, the Academy established a new designation: Fellow of the Academy of Nutrition and Dietetics (FAND). This honor recognizes Academy leadership, volunteer, and presentation experience on behalf of the Association. Recipients add the designation "FAND" to their title.

Several other honors and awards are given annually in recognition of outstanding service at the state or national level and for leadership in specific areas of practice. The Academy also recognizes one or more persons in allied professions by bestowing honorary membership. The Honors Committee of the Board of Directors establishes criteria for the awards and makes selections among those nominated for national awards.

DIETETICS AS A PROFESSION

A *profession* is defined as an area of practice with the following characteristics: specialized knowledge, continuing education, a code of ethics, and a commitment to service for others. Plato first described a profession as "the occupation ... to which one devotes himself, a calling in which one professes to have acquired some special knowledge used by way of instruction, guidance, or advice to others, or of servicing them in some art."[20] Dietetics, like other professions that fit Plato's description, is organized around these principles in the following ways:

Specialized knowledge. Standards for education for dietetics were established as early as 1919. At least 2 years of college was first recommended, which later became a 4-year requirement or a 2-year course for institutional managers. Courses for the bachelor's degree were specified, and, later, hospital training of 6 months was added to the educational requirement. Subsequent education plans were introduced that continued to specify needed courses. In 1987, standards of education were established, by which dietetics education focused more on the outcomes of the educational process. The ADA set up a review process that periodically updated educational requirements as the profession grew and matured. Dietitians and employers alike recognize the specialized knowledge required to practice in dietetics.

Continuing education. When dietetics was registered as an accredited profession in the 1960s, a requirement of 75 hours of continuing education each 5 years was initiated. A wide number of educational events were recognized as meeting this requirement and were given credit accordingly.

Continuing professional education is a well-established function of the Academy through the center for professional education, which offers conferences, annual meeting events, and other opportunities.

A code of ethics. A code of ethics for its members was developed in 1942.[21] The code was updated and expanded over the years, moving from the *Code of Professional Conduct* to the 2009 *Code of Ethics for the Profession of Dietetics and Process for Consideration of Ethics Issues.* Published jointly by the Academy and the Commission on Dietetic Registration, it provides guidance to dietetic practitioners in their professional practice and conduct.[22]

Service to others. The seal of the Academy carries the motto, "Quam Plurimis Prodesse," which means, "benefit as many as possible." Dietitians recognize a professional commitment to help the public attain optimal health and quality of life through the practice of good nutritional habits. The organization reflects this imperative in all areas of practice.

As of January 1, 2012, the name of the association was changed to the Academy of Nutrition and Dietetics.

GROWTH OF THE PROFESSION

Membership

In 1917, the requirements for membership were lenient to bring in as many practitioners as possible. Gradually, however, active membership became based on specified education and practical experience. Several categories of membership have been added over the years, and at present, the categories are active, honorary, international, retired, student, and associate members.

Membership in the Academy has risen steadily over the years. The membership grew by about 1000 to 1500 each decade until a growth spurt in the late 1960s, with the addition of about 15,000 members between 1968 and 1978. In 2015, the membership stood over 75,000 of which about 5 percent were men.

Registration and Licensure

In 1969, the association established the system of national professional certification under which the dietitian was designated as a registered dietitian (RD). The title carried legal status and denoted the professional who met the education and experience requirements to practice, in addition to participating in continuing education, thereby maintaining currency of practice. A national testing program was also developed to establish eligibility. Employers soon became familiar with the RD credential and began specifying it as a condition of employment. Today, 75 percent of all dietitians are registered.

Licensure of dietitians occurs in states in which state governments have passed legislation recognizing the profession and awarded state-level legal standing. Forty-seven states have enacted licensure laws for dietitians.

The Academy of Nutrition and Dietetics Foundation

The arm of the association with a tax status identifying it as an educational and scientific nonprofit organization, the Foundation solicits and accepts monies donated for scholarships, research, and other designated projects. Several major studies have been funded by the foundation, and programs and lectureships at the annual meeting have been made possible through gifts and donations.

Dietetic Technicians and Managers

Managers. The Hospital, Institution, and Educational Food Service Society (HIEFSS) was formed in 1960 as an organization for food service supervisors. It was an independent society but closely tied to the ADA through membership standards as well as financial support. The name was later changed to the Association for Managers of Food Operations (AMFO), and the title for members became food manager. The current name of this association is the Association of Nutrition and Foodservice Professionals (ANFP). Persons completing a voluntary certificate program have the title, certified dietary manager (CDA). Membership stands at over 14,000.

Dietetic technicians. Dietetic technician programs require specific education and training, usually 2 years in a community college program of study. As with the RD, the technician member can also become registered by meeting the specific standards and passing an examination. He or she earns the title dietetic technician, registered (DTR).

Several milestones in the history of the DTRs follow:[23]

- *1986.* The American Dietetic Association grandfathered 3618 dietetic technicians into membership.
- *1987.* The first administration of the registration exam for dietetic technicians in nutrition care services and food service systems management was conducted.

- *1987.* The passing standard for the registration examination for dietetic technicians was established.
- *1988.* Continuing education requirements for DTRs were enacted.
- *1990.* First DTR elected to the Commission on Dietetic Registration.
- *1990.* Administration of the first registration examination based on the 1990 role delineation study took place, and new passing standards were developed.
- *1996.* New test specifications for the DTR examination were implemented.
- *2007.* New test specifications for DTR registration examination were implemented.
- *2009.* Pathway III process was implemented to allow didactic program in dietetics graduates to sit for the DTR examination.
- *2015.* Membership stood at 75,000.

Legislative Activity

Involvement in legislative activity began when dietitians promoted a bill to grant military rank to dietitians serving in World War I. In the 1940s and 1950s, legislative activity centered around setting standards for employment in the Veterans Administration, passage of the national School Lunch Act, and, in 1946, support of the Maternal and Child Health bill. Signaling even more extensive efforts, the association changed its tax status in the 1960s to permit active lobbying and made its voice heard by establishing an office in Washington, DC, and taking positions on national issues. A political action committee (PAC) was formed in 1980, through which Academy members donate funds and recognize legislators who promote legislation on behalf of food and nutrition issues. Each year, the Academy identifies key legislative issues for particular attention and activity by the Washington office and members. The current legislative priorities for the Academy are discussed later in this chapter.

Areas of Practice

The practice of dietetics was first structured around four areas in which dietitians were employed. Little was documented about the number of dietitians working in each area until periodic membership surveys were initiated in the early 1980s. As shown in **Table 1-1**, clinical dietetics is the area in which the highest number of dietitians work. Fifty-six percent

Table 1-1. Primary Area of Practice by Dietitians (Percent)

Practice Area	2007[a]	2009[b]	2011[c]	2013[d]	2015[e]
Clinical dietetics	55	56	56	57	57
Food and nutrition management	12	12	12	12	11
Community nutrition	11	11	11	11	10
Consultation/business	11	8	8	8	8
Education/research	6	7	7	6	7
Other	5	6	6	6	7

Sources: a. Rogers, D. "Compensation and Benefits Survey 2007: Above Average Pay Gain Seen for Registered Dietitians." *J Am Diet Assoc* 108 (2008): 416–425.

b. American Dietetic Association. Compensation and Benefits Survey of the Dietetics Profession 2009. Accessed October 20, 2009, www.eatright.org

c. Warde, B. "Compensation and Benefits Survey 2011: Moderate Growth in Registered Dietitian and Dietetic Technician Registered, Compensation in the Past 2 Years." *J Acad Nutr Diet* 112 (2012): 29–40.

d. Rogers, D. "Compensation and Benefits Survey 2013: Education and Job Responsibility Key to Increased Compensation." *J Acad Nutr Diet* 113 (2014):17–33.

e. Rogers, D. "Compensation and Benefits Survey 2015." *J Acad Nutr Diet* 116, no. 3 (2016): 370–388.

of DTRs also work in clinical practice. Although this initially designated hospital-related dietetics, the clinical dietetics category now includes acute inpatient, ambulatory, and long-term care. The number of dietitians working in food service administration has declined in recent years while other areas of practice have remained close to the same.

Dietetic Practice Groups

Dietetic practice groups (DPGs) are formed by Academy members practicing in or having a particular interest in an identified area of practice. DPGs provide a means of networking among group members. The groups elect officers, collect dues, and publish a newsletter or similar communication for its members. From the original 9 groups established in 1978, there are now 26 practice groups.[24] Additional subgroups, or member interest groups (MIGs), have also been formed.

Long-Range Planning

Leaders in dietetics have consistently taken steps to position the profession to meet both present and future needs. This has been achieved through planning groups, task forces, committees, and outside consultants. In 1959, through a study, it was determined that active recruitment, educational opportunities, interaction with other professional groups, and an emphasis on research were needed for continued growth and development of the profession. These goals were expanded in the 1970s with the appointment of a task force and a study commission on dietetics. The study outcome was a report that examined the roles of dietitians and their educational needs for the future. Titled, *The Profession of Dietetics: The Report of the Study Commission on Dietetics*, the report influenced the direction of the association for many years. A second in-depth study in 1984 became a major reference source for long-range planning.[25,26]

Many planning activities that moved the profession forward in significant ways were initiated in the 1980s. The first of a series of long-range planning conferences convened in 1981, with a second in 1984. Invited leaders discussed goals and needs and made far-reaching recommendations. The future was also explored in a strategic planning conference in 1995.[27] The ADA moved decisively toward public outreach and increased involvement in the policy arena, although emphasis on association members and their professional welfare continued.

Further landmark studies examined the education of dietitians, registration and licensure, and advanced practice. In the 1970s, a master plan for education for practice identified trends affecting the demand for dietitians and estimated numbers that would be needed in the future.[28] Role delineation studies included dietetic technicians and described the roles of dietitians and technicians in a variety of settings. These and other studies in the 1990s, including one by the Task Force on Critical Issues: Registration Eligibility and Licensure,[29] continued to show opportunities that enhanced both education and practice and led to continued advances in the profession.

Two task forces in early 2000, the Task Force on the Future Practice and Education and the Phase 2, Future Practice and Education Task Force, initiated broad and comprehensive studies of practice and education.[30]

The board of directors undertakes long-range planning on a regular basis. Using expert consultants and the results of special studies and surveys, the board examines trends impacting dietetic practice to make long-term projections and set goals. The *Strategic Plan of 2011–2012* is the current document outlining the association's goals.

Professional Partnerships

The Academy currently maintains liaisons with some 140 allied groups and associations. The formation of these partnerships has advanced mutual efforts and made many programs and activities possible. A long-standing affiliation with the American Public Health Association and the American Diabetes Association has resulted in the development of the diabetic exchange lists and joint publication of the booklet, *Choose Your Foods: Exchange Lists for Diabetes*. Grants from the public health association also allowed the ADA to sponsor workshops on programmed learning. The U.S. Public Health Service sponsors a nutrition section that administers programs critical to health care in the United States. The American Diabetes Association exchanges speakers with the Academy at conferences and annual meetings.

The American Hospital Association is another important organization allied with the Academy. Hospitals employ many dietitians who contribute to patient care. Hospital-accrediting bodies (e.g., the Joint Commission) include nutrition and food services in their surveys regarding the quality of the services.

The Food and Nutrition Science Alliance (FANSA) was formed in 1992 with the Institute of Food Technology, the American Society for Clinical Nutrition, and the American Society of Nutritional Science. This linkage brought together a combined membership of more than 100,000 who join forces to speak with one voice on food and nutrition issues and to translate scientific information into practical advice for consumers. FANSA is a partnership of seven professional scientific societies whose members have joined forces to speak with one voice on food and nutrition issues.[31]

The Academy of Nutrition and Dietetics has participated in many programs with governmental agencies, including the U.S. Department of Agriculture (USDA), the Department of Health and Human Services (DHHS), the National Institutes of Health, the National Research Council, and the U.S. Congress.

The International Confederation of Dietetic Associations is composed of 34 national dietetic associations. The American Dietetic Association was an early member of this group. The purposes of the confederation are to achieve integrated communication; promote an enhanced image for the profession; and increase awareness of standards of education, training, and practice in dietetics.

The American Overseas Academy is affiliated with the Academy. The members are Academy members living overseas. The members enjoy the same benefits and privileges as other Academy of Nutrition and Dietetics–affiliated groups.

An International Congress of Dietetics is held in a major city every 5 years. The first congress was held in Amsterdam in 1952, with the ADA as one of the founding groups. Organized for the purpose of sharing information, the congress publishes an international bulletin and holds an annual meeting. The 2012 congress was held in Sydney, Australia.

REACHING OUT TO THE PUBLIC

The Academy has initiated many programs over the years directed to the general public. Foremost among the services currently offered by the organization are the Academy website, www.eatright.org, and toll-free number, 1-800-877-1600. The website is a source of current information for professionals as well as consumers interested in food and nutrition issues and programs. Employers searching for a dietitian may also use the website to make connections.

Begun as a Dietitian's Week observance in three states, this focus is now a month-long event each March with both local and national emphasis and known as *National Nutrition Month.*

A dial-a-dietitian program, funded by the Nutrition Foundation, was started in Detroit in 1961. Many states now offer similar services designed to provide information in a timely manner in response to questions from the public.

A training program was initiated in 1982 to prepare selected dietitians to serve as spokespersons for the profession to reach the public with food and nutrition information through the media. More spokespersons, including state media persons, have been added in most major media in the United States. Referred to as the spokesperson network, the program continues to be highly successful at reaching the public with timely and reliable information through television and other media outlets.

Participation in national projects and campaigns is another way the association impacts the public. Over the years, campaigns on women's health, child nutrition, osteoporosis, high blood pressure, and other issues have been the focus of several medical and health-related groups, including the Academy.

Childhood obesity has been a focus of the Academy and the Foundation for several years in concert with other governmental and private groups, such as The Alliance for a Healthier Generation. Academy members also serve on the committee to develop the Dietary Guidelines for Americans and on the Food and Nutrition Board of the National Academy of Sciences.

HISTORICAL EVENTS IN THE ACADEMY OF NUTRITION AND DIETETICS

A series of historical events in the association have been published beginning in 2012. The titles are as follows:

- History and Governance[32]
- Networking Groups[33]
- The Foundation[34]
- Dietetic Students[35]
- The Military Roots[36]
- Corporate Relations[37]
- The Academy's Past[38]
- Annual Meeting[39]
- Founding of the Academy[40]
- Recruitment Materials[41]
- Communications[42]
- Modern History[43]

SUMMARY

The history of the dietetics profession is a rich account of consistent growth, forward-thinking leaders, and the emergence of dietitians as leaders among those concerned with the health and well-being of all citizens. As a profession, dietetics has established standards for practitioner education, a code of ethics, registration and licensure systems, and a tradition of partnership and collaboration with others in allied areas of professional practice to extend outreach and service. The Academy of Nutrition and

Dietetics supports its members as they practice in a wide variety of careers, and it also reaches out to the public with timely and reliable information about food and nutrition issues.

DEFINITIONS

Academy of Nutrition and Dietetics. The professional organization for dietitians. Formerly known as the *American Dietetic Association.*

Dietetic practice group (DPG). An organized group of Academy of Nutrition and Dietetics members with similar interests in an area of practice or a particular subject area.

Dietetic technician. A graduate of an approved dietetic technician program.

Dietitian. A professional who translates the science of food and nutrition to enhance the health and well-being of individuals and groups.

Nutritionist. A professional with academic credentials in nutrition; he or she may also be an RD.

Registered dietitian (RD). A dietitian who has fulfilled the eligibility requirements of the Commission on Dietetic Registration.

REFERENCES

1. Barber, M.I. *History of the American Dietetic Association (1917–1959).* (Philadelphia: JB Lippincott Co., 1959), p. 3.
2. Corbett, F.R. "The Training of Dietitians for Hospitals." *J Home Ec* 1 (1909): 62.
3. ADA. *A New Look at the Profession of Dietetics. Report of the 1984 Study Commission on Dietetics.* (Chicago: The American Dietetic Association, 1985), p. 29.
4. Todhunter, E.N. "Development of Knowledge in Nutrition. 1. Animal Experiments." *J Am Diet Assoc* 41 (1962): 328–334.
5. Beeuwkes, A.M. "The Prevalence of Scurvy among Voyageurs to America 1493–1600." *J Am Diet Assoc* 24 (1948): 300–304.
6. Goldberger, J. "Pellagra." *J Am Diet Assoc* 4 (1929): 212–227.
7. McCoy, C.M. "Seven Centuries of Scientific Nutrition." *J Am Diet Assoc* 15 (1939): 648–658.
8. Shircliffe, A. "American Schools of Cookery." *J Am Diet Assoc* 23 (1947): 776–777.
9. See Note 3.
10. Rorer, S.T. "Early Dietetics." *J Am Diet Assoc* 10 (1934): 289–295.
11. Cassell, J. *Carry the Flame: The History of the American Dietetic Association.* (Chicago: The American Dietetic Association, 1990).

12. Cooper, L.F. "Florence Nightingale's Contribution to Dietetics." *J Am Diet Assoc* 39 (1954): 121–127.
13. Mathieu, J. "RDs in the Military." *J Am Diet Assoc* 108, no. 12 (2008): 1984–1987.
14. See Note 11.
15. See Note 3.
16. See Note 11.
17. Ibid.
18. Ibid.
19. President's Page. "Members Who Have Climbed to the Top." *J Acad Nutr Diet* 114, no. 4 (2014): 517.
20. See Note 11.
21. Ibid.
22. American Dietetic Association/Commission on Dietetic Registration. "Code of Ethics for the Profession of Dietetics and Process for Consideration of Ethics Issues." *J Am Diet Assoc* 109, no. 8 (2009): 1461–1467.
23. Babjak, P. Personal communication.
24. List of Dietetic Practice Groups (DPGs). www.eatright.org (10/11/15)
25. ADA. *The Profession of Dietetics. The Report of the Study Commission on Dietetics.* (Chicago: The American Dietetic Association, 1972).
26. "A new look at the profession of dietetics. Final report of the American Dietetic Association Foundation 1984 Study Commission on Dietetics: Summary and recommendations." *J Am Diet Assoc* 84 (1984): 1052–1063.
27. ADA. *ADA Annual Report. 1994–1995.* (Chicago: The American Dietetic Association, 1995), p. 5.
28. Council on Educational Preparation. "Report of the Task Force on Competencies." *J Am Diet Assoc* 73 (1978): 281.
29. Registration Eligibility and Licensure Task Force. *Report of the Critical Issues.* (Chicago: The American Dietetic Association, 1992).
30. ADA. *Report of the Phase 2. Future Practice and Education Task Force.* (Chicago: American Dietetic Association, 2008).
31. Food and Nutrition Service Alliance. www.foodprocessding.com/industrylinks.
32. Stein, K. "The Academy's Governance and Practice: Restructuring for the Challenges of the Turn of the 21st Century." *J Acad Nutr Diet* 112, no. 11 (2012): 1871–1896.
33. Stein, K. "Networking Groups: Advancing Nutrition and Practice Groups through Practice, Culture, and Geography." *J Acad Nutr Diet* 113, no. 2 (2013): 326–343.
34. Stein, K. "Advancing the Dietetics Profession through the Foundation's Philanthropy." *J Acad Nutr Diet* 113, no. 6 (2013): 834–855.
35. Stein, K. "History Snapshot: Dietetics Student Experience in the 1940s." *J Acad Nutr Diet* 114, no. 10 (2014): 1648–1662.
36. Stein, K. "The Academy's Military Roots Visualized." *J Acad Nutr Diet* 114, no. 12 (2014): 2023–2049.

37. Stein, K. "Advancing Health through Sustained Collaboration: How the History of Corporate Relations Extended the Academy's Reach." *J Acad Nutr Diet* 115, no. 1 (2015): 131–142.

38. Stein, K. "What We Ate: Reports of the Academy's Past." *J Acad Nutr Diet* 115, no. 2 (2015): 286–302.

39. Stein, K. "Coming Together Conference: A Philosophic Journey through Academy Annual Meeting in the 20th Century." *J Acad Nutr Diet* 115, no. 4 (2015): 635–659.

40. Stein, K. "A Few Days in Autumn: The Founding of the Academy of Nutrition and Dietetics." *J Acad Nutr Diet* 115, no. 6 (2015): 1008–1009.

41. Stein, K. "A Pictorial Job Fair: A Glimpse at the Academy's Vintage Professional Recruitment Materials." *J Acad Nutr Diet* 115, no. 9 (2015): 1500–1513.

42. Stein, K. "Communications at the Academy: Where Strategy and Trending Conspire to Shape History." *J Acad Nutr Diet* 115, no. 7 (2015): 1148–1168.

43. Stein, K. "The Value of Belonging: The Recent History of Member Services at the Academy." *J Acad Nutr Diet* 116, no. 1 (2016): 100–162.

CHAPTER 2

The Academy of Nutrition and Dietetics

"Our capacity to influence the public—to *change lives*—is limitless, and it is something we do year-round."[1]

OUTLINE

- Learning Objectives
- Introduction
- The Strategic Plan
- Membership Categories
- Membership Benefits
- Governance of the Academy of Nutrition and Dietetics
  - Board of Directors
  - House of Delegates
  - Accreditation Council for Education in Nutrition and Dietetics
  - Commission on Dietetic Registration
  - Dietetic Practice Groups
- Position Papers
- Dietitian Salaries
- Affiliated Units of the Academy of Nutrition and Dietetics
  - State and District Associations
  - Academy of Nutrition and Dietetics Foundation
  - Washington Office
  - American Overseas Dietetic Association

- Summary
- Definitions
- References

LEARNING OBJECTIVES

The student will be able to:

1. Name and describe the functions of the various governing groups in the Academy.
2. Become familiar with dietetic practice groups (DPGs) and their purposes.
3. Know the categories of membership and their requirements.
4. Understand how goals and priorities are part of a strategic plan for an organization.
5. Discuss member benefits.

INTRODUCTION

The Academy of Nutrition and Dietetics stands as the professional organization of about 75,000 food and nutrition experts (5 percent male and 95 percent female). In the 99 years since its founding, this organization has been the major forum for the networking of dietitians, for research related to food and nutrition, for managerial activities, and for political activities necessary to govern itself and for outreach to the public.

The original constitution and bylaws of the association have been amended frequently, but the focus of the association has remained constant from the beginning: maintaining a concern for the continuing interests of dietitians and dietetic professionals in their education, practice opportunities, and research for the future. The Academy, as the professional association for practitioners, has long-standing concerns for the protection of the public in areas of nutritional health and disease prevention and the welfare of the practitioner (or individual member). The organization and its leaders of elected members have worked through the years to keep these concerns in focus.

The mission statement of the Academy of Nutrition and Dietetics is, "empowering members to be the nation's food and nutrition leaders."[2] The mission statement sets the agenda for the association and its programs and is described as the association's reason for being. The values that guide the organizational and member behavior are *customer focus, integrity, innovation, social responsibility*, and *diversity*.[3] The values are defined as:

Customer focus—meet the needs and exceed the expectations of all customers.

Integrity—act ethically with accountability for lifelong learning, commitment to excellence, and professionalism.

Innovation—embrace change with creativity and strategic thinking.

Social responsibility—make decisions with consideration for inclusivity as well as environmental, economic, and social implications.

Diversity—recognize and respect differences in culture, ethnicity, age, gender, race, creed, religion, sexual orientation, physical ability, politics, and socioeconomic characteristics.

The vision of the Academy is to "optimize the nation's health through food and nutrition."[4]

THE STRATEGIC PLAN

Through activation of the mission and vision statements along with the identified values and goals, a strategic plan for the Academy and its members is in effect. The goals help focus, set priorities, and assign resources. They specify outcomes and represent what needs to be achieved. Four major goals are identified along with 16 strategies to help define how the goals are to be accomplished.[5] The goals are:

1. The public trusts and chooses Registered Dietitian/Nutritionists as food, nutrition and health experts.
2. Academy members optimize the health of individuals and populations served.
3. Members and prospective members view the Academy as vital to professional success.
4. Members collaborate across disciplines with international and nutrition communities.

In 2008, the Academy adopted a standard logo, replacing a mix of over 100 different visual brands.[6] The logo bears the words, "Eat right."

MEMBERSHIP CATEGORIES

Membership in the Academy is available in any one of the following categories: active, honorary, retired, student, international.[7] Associate membership is also available to practitioners in other fields.

The largest category of membership is *active*, which generally includes those who hold a baccalaureate degree and have met academic requirements specified by the Academy; an individual with an advanced degree and an emphasis in a closely allied area with dietetics; or a dietetic technician, registered (DTR). In addition, any person who has completed a term as president of the association or one who has previously paid dues to obtain life membership may also hold active membership.

The *retired* member category is an option for any member who is at least 62 years of age, either actively employed or no longer employed. *Student* members are those enrolled in an accredited program, a student in a college degree program intending to enter an accredited program, or active members returning to school for a degree in a dietetic-related course of study. *Honorary* membership is awarded to individuals who have made contributions to the field of nutrition or dietetics and are deemed eligible by the board of directors (BOD). *International* members are those persons who have completed formal training outside the United States and U.S. territories and have been verified by a country's professional dietetics association or regulatory body. The *Associate* category is open to persons in allied fields with a minimum of a bachelor's degree and training or certification in a specified profession. See the Academy website for a listing of the designated professions.

The rights and privileges of each of the membership categories appear in the bylaws of the Academy. The dues may change from year to year by action of the house of delegates (HOD). Dues differ for each category, with a portion of the national dues offsetting the cost of the *Journal of the Academy of Nutrition and Dietetics* and a rebate returned to the state affiliate associations for each member of the state. In addition, the national dietetic practice groups (DPGs) charge for membership in their groups and provide newsletters and other educational materials for members in the specific practice area.

MEMBERSHIP BENEFITS

Membership in the Academy benefits the individual and collective members in many ways.[8] These may be summarized under the following categories:

- Websites
- Publications and subscriptions
- Career resources
- Practice resources
- Social networking
- Educational opportunities
- Policy initiatives and advocacy
- Science and quality
- Networking and promotions
- Promotional resources
- Branding services
- Additional benefits
- Honors and awards
- Professional insurance
- Academy Credit Card

GOVERNANCE OF THE ACADEMY OF NUTRITION AND DIETETICS

The organizational structure of the ADA/Academy of Nutrition and Dietetics changed over time; however, governance has been through members who were either elected, appointed, or volunteered from the membership at large. Those elected each year are the officers serving on the BOD, delegates to the HOD by states, members of the Commission on Dietetic Registration, and members of the Accreditation Council for Education in Nutrition and Dietetics (ACEND). Members of the foundation board are appointed, and membership in DPGs is by member choice. A chief executive officer (CEO) is employed by the board to oversee and manage a paid staff at the headquarters in Chicago. Under the leadership of the CEO, the staff members form partnerships with the various volunteer groups, forming teams to accomplish the variety of tasks necessary to keep the organization functional and to implement the strategic plan. The BOD and the HOD function as a voice for members.

Board of Directors

The board of directors (BOD) is composed of 19 members: president, president-elect, past president, treasurer, treasurer-elect, past treasurer, three directors at large, six HOD directors, two public members, the foundation chair, and the CEO, who is nonvoting. The BOD governs the organization through the following activities:

- Sets and monitors strategic direction
- Oversees fiscal planning
- Provides leadership for professional initiatives
- Selects, supports, and assesses the CEO and conducts an annual performance appraisal
- Appoints persons to represent the association
- Establishes guidelines and policies for appeals, publications, awards, and honors
- Administers and enforces the professional code of ethics
- Exercises powers and performs lawful acts under the Illinois Not-for-Profit Corporation Act

House of Delegates

The house of delegates (HOD) is composed of 105 delegates who represent each state, almost all the DPGs, the Commission of Dietetic Registration, ACEND, dietetic technicians, and student members. The House leadership team develops and implements program goals of the House. Issues that are identified as important to the membership are discussed at each Spring and Fall session of the HOD.

The House of Delegates includes 105 members as follows:

- 66 Affiliate Delegates elected by members of the 53 affiliate dietetic associations.
- 26 Dietetic Practice Group (DPG) members elected or appointed by each DPG
- 7 at-large Delegates as follows: 1 from ACEND, 1 from CDR, 1 student member, 1 under age 30 member, 1 from DTR, 1 retired member, and 1 from NDEP.
- 6 HOD Directors including the Speaker, Speaker-elect, immediate past speaker, 3 appointed

The House of Delegates, as the voice of members, governs the profession and develops policy on many professional issues.

The Leadership team develops and implements programs based on the core functions as follows:

- Member focus
- Information systems and communications
- Strategic thinking and visioning
- New products and services development
- Governance
- Professional leadership
- Setting policy for the profession
- Financial

The HOD provides a forum for membership and professional issues, and establishes and maintains professional standards of the membership. Core roles of the HOD include adopting and maintaining a code of ethics in conjunction with the CDR, developing position statements and other professional papers, establishing qualifications and dues of members, and the formula for dues payment to affiliate organizations. The HOD also identifies and prioritizes trends and recommends policy and strategic direction for the Academy. The HOD has the authority to establish committees and rules and policies of organization and governance, including its own composition and size.

Both the BOD and the HOD represent Academy members and govern the Academy. As a comparison, the BOD is likened to the executive branch of the U.S. government and the HOD to the legislative branch. Both groups work together closely to promote the interests of the members and further the profession.

Accreditation Council for Education in Nutrition and Dietetics

The Accreditation Council for Education in Nutrition and Dietetics (ACEND) establishes and enforces standards for the educational preparation of dietetics professionals and recognizes dietetics education programs that meet the standards. The ACEND administers and has authority for all actions that apply to accreditation of entry-level education programs that include standard setting, fees, finances, and administration. There are 12 members on the council. At least half of the members represent each program type (dietetic technician, didactic, coordinated, and dietetic internship). The council includes one representative of other constituents, one dietetic student, and two representatives of the public.

Commission on Dietetic Registration

The mission of the Commission on Dietetic Registration (CDR) is to protect the public through credentialing and assessment procedures that ensure the competence of registered dietitians and dietetic technicians, registered and specialists.

The CDR sets the standards for certification and recertification and enforces the code of ethics of the association. The commission issues credentials to those individuals who meet the standards. Dietitians thus attain the registered dietitian (RD) designation, and dietetic technicians, the DTR. Specialists receive the certified specialist title.

Dietetic Practice Groups

Dietetic practice groups (DPGs) are professional interest groups within the Academy framework. The 28 active groups show the diversity of the practice areas in which dietitians work (**Table 2-1**). Each group networks to serve its members, charges fees to support its activities, and maintains communication with its members by various means. The groups also sponsor educational sessions at the annual meeting. The requirements to join a DPG are Academy membership or registration status and payment of dues. A member may belong to as many groups as desired.

Formation of new groups occurs after interest groups become large enough to seek official status. A petition is submitted with no fewer than 500 signatures indicating interest, individuals willing to serve as officers, and a budget. Aside from maintaining a minimum of 300 members, other uniform requirements include publication of a newsletter at least quarterly for its members, maintaining governing documents, conducting an annual meeting of its members, and maintaining a balanced budget. DPGs offer networking opportunities with professionals with similar interests and provide significant opportunities for leadership responsibilities both within the DPG and the Academy.

A practice group may also develop subunits or groups of members within the DPG based on a practice area or issue of interest to the members of the group, thus creating an even smaller group of dietitians with closely allied interests. Currently, 30 subspecialty areas exist within the

Table 2-1.   Dietetic Practice Groups 2015–2016

2015–2016 Dietetic Practice Groups (DPGs)	Description
Behavioral Health Nutrition (BHN) DPG	BHN members are the most valued source of food and nutrition service for persons with addictions, eating disorders, intellectual and developmental disabilities, and mental illness.
Clinical Nutrition Management (CNM) DPG	Managers who direct clinical nutrition programs across the continuum of care.
Diabetes Care and Education (DCE) DPG	Members involved in patient and professional education, as well as research for the management of diabetes.
Dietetic Technicians in Practice (DTP) DPG	Members are advocates for dietetic technician, registered, as dietetics practitioners in providing quality client care.
Dietitians in Health Care Communities (DHCC) DPG	Practitioners typically employed under contract who provide nutrition consultation to acute and long-term-care facilities, home care companies, healthcare agencies, and the foodservice industry.
Dietitians in Business and Communications (DBC) DPG	Food and nutrition practitioners who work for or consult with corporations, businesses, and organizations, or who are self-employed or business owners.
Dietitians in Integrative and Functional Medicine (DIFM) DPG	Food and nutrition practitioners that promote the integration of conventional nutrition practices with evidenced-based alternatives including functional and integrative medicine and nutrition.
Dietitians in Nutrition Support (DNS) DPG	Dietitians who integrate the science and practice of enteral and parenteral nutrition to provide nutrition support therapy to individuals (adults, pediatrics, inpatients, outpatients, home care, transplantation, and complex gastrointestinal disorders).
Food and Culinary Professionals (FCP) DPG	Members who promote food education and culinary skills to enhance quality of life and health of the public.
Healthy Aging (HA) DPG	Practitioners who provide and manage nutrition programs and services to older adults in a variety of settings.
Hunger and Environmental Nutrition (HEN) DPG	Members who lead the future in sustainable and accessible food and water systems through education, research, and action.
Management in Food and Nutrition Systems (MFNS) DPG	Food and nutrition care managers generally employed in healthcare institution, universities, corrections, and other facilities.

(continues)

Table 2-1.   Dietetic Practice Groups 2015–2016 (Continued)

2015–2016 Dietetic Practice Groups (DPGs)	Description
Medical Nutrition Practice Group (MNPG) DPG	Practitioners who practice a wide range of medical nutrition therapy across the continuum of care in a variety of settings.
Nutrition Education for the Public (NEP) DPG	Practitioners involved in the design, implementation, and evaluation of nutrition education programs for target populations.
Nutrition Educators of Health Professionals (NEHP) DPG	Members involved in education and communication with physicians, nurses, dentists, and other healthcare professionals.
Nutrition Entrepreneurs (NE) DPG	NE members shape the future of dietetics practice by pursuing innovative and creative ways of providing nutrition products and services to consumers, industry, media, and business.
Oncology Nutrition (ON) DPG	Members shape the future of dietetics practice by pursuing innovative and creative ways to provide nutrition products and services to consumer, industry, media, and business.
Pediatric Nutrition (PNPG) DPG	Practitioners who provide nutrition services for the pediatric population in a wide variety of settings.
Public Health/Community Nutrition (PHCNPG) DPG	Nutrition professionals who work in partnership with healthcare providers, community leaders, and other key stakeholders to serve the public in a variety of roles and settings.
Renal Dietitians (RPG) DPG	Practitioners who provide medical nutrition service to chronic kidney disease patients in dialysis facilities, clinics, hospitals, university settings, and private practice.
Research (RDPG) DPG	Members who conduct research in various areas to promote practice standards, health policy, and disease prevention.
School Nutrition Services (SNS) DPG	School foodservice directors, nutrition educators, and corporate dietitians working in the delivery of food service and nutrition education to children.
Sports, Cardiovascular, and Wellness Nutrition (SCAN) DPG	Nutrition practitioners with expertise and skills in promoting the role of nutrition in physical performance, cardiovascular health, wellness, and disordered eating.
Vegetarian Nutrition (VN) DPG	Nutrition practitioners who focus on information and resources for plant-based diets.

Table 2-1.   Dietetic Practice Groups 2015–2016 (Continued)

2015–2016 Dietetic Practice Groups (DPGs)	Description
Weight Management (WM) DPG	Practitioners who work in the prevention and treatment of overweight and obesity throughout the life cycle.
Women's Health (WH) DPG	Practitioners addressing women's nutrition care issues during the reproductive period through menopause.

Printed with permission from Academy of Nutrition and Dietetics.

main DPGs. In addition, 10 Member Interest Groups (MIGs) have been formed whereby specific population groups can share mutual interests. (See www.eatright.org for lists of sub groups and member interest groups.)

POSITION PAPERS

A position paper represents a consensus of viewpoints and professional interests and is used in many ways such as in media contacts, in drafting legislation and testifying before governmental groups, and for communication with the public. A nutrition position paper is described as a statement of the association's stance on an issue that affects the nutritional status of the public; it is derived from pertinent facts and data, and is germane to the Academy's mission, vision, philosophy, and values. Position papers are periodically updated or deleted, and others added by the HOD. Copies of current position papers are available from the Academy headquarters office or at www.eatright.org.

DIETITIAN SALARIES

The salary levels of dietitians and dietetic technicians have risen over the years, with certain practice areas commanding higher salaries. These changes reflect the increasingly important roles played by dietitians and dietetic technicians. In 1938, it was reported that hospital dietitians, on the average, earned an annual salary in the range of $1090 to $7000. At that time, benefits such as room, board, and laundry were often supplied by the employer in addition to a salary. In positions other than those offered by hospitals, the salaries ranged from $1200 to $4000 per year.

In 1946, the average salary was reported to be $3000—not a significant improvement.[9]

In 1981, the ADA initiated the first survey of members that reported salaries along with other data regarding employment. At that time, the average yearly salary was $16,000, although the study did not equate all salaries with full-time practice and the actual full-time salaries were probably higher.[10] The median yearly salary for dietitians in all areas of practice from 2007 to 2015 is shown in **Table 2-2**. In 2015, the median salary for all dietitians was $63,700.

When comparing salaries by areas of practice in dietetics, it is apparent that dietitians in food and nutrition management and education/research have the highest incomes while those earning the least are in community nutrition practice. Several factors account for differences in compensation: years in a position, education level, job responsibilities, number of persons supervised, budget responsibility, and location.[11]

Table 2-2.   Median Income for Registered Dietitians by Area of Practice

Practice Area	2007[a]	2009[b]	2011[c]	2013[d]	2015[e]
Clinical	51,668	55,390	56,056	58,280	60,320
Food and nutrition management	64,002	67,995	70,990	74,006	78,000
Community nutrition	48,006	52,000	51,120	54,205	56,000
Consultation/business	60,008	69,992	65,000	65,603	77,000
Education/research	66,061	65,000	64,000	65,000	80,000
All areas	53,000	56,700	57,990	60,000	63,700

Sources: a. Rogers, D. "Compensation and Benefits Survey 2007: Above-Average Pay Gain Seen for Registered Dietitians." *J Am Diet Assoc* 108 (2008): 446–425.

b. American Dietetic Association. "Compensation and Benefits Survey of the Dietetics Profession 2009," accessed at www.eatright.org.

c. Ward, B. "Compensation and Benefits Survey 2011: Moderate Growth in Registered Dietitian and Dietetic Technician, Registered, Compensation in the Past 2 Years." *J Acad Nutr Diet* 1 (2012): 29–40.

d. Rogers, D. "Compensation and Benefits Survey 2013: Education and Job Responsibility Key to Increased Compensation." *J Acad Nutr Diet* 114, no. 1 (2014): 17–33

e. Rogers, D. "Compensation and Benefits Survey." *J Acad Nutr Diet* 116, no. 3 (2016): 370–388.

The median wage for the registered dietetic technician was $36,000 in 2007, $39,000 in 2009, $40,000 in 2011, $40,000 in 2013, and $43,000 in 2015.[12]

AFFILIATED UNITS OF THE ACADEMY OF NUTRITION AND DIETETICS

State and District Associations

Each of the 50 states and Puerto Rico are affiliates of the Academy and are organized with state and district associations. Membership in the Academy determines the membership in state affiliates because states generally charge no membership fees and instead receive rebates from the Academy according to the number of members. A member of the Academy is automatically a member of a state affiliate.

The state organizations for the most are parallel to the national organization. Each state elects its delegates to represent its members in the HOD. The number of district organizations is determined by the states as well as how they fit into the state organization. The district groups provide educational and informational programs for the grassroots members. Most states have one or two meetings per year that provide continuing education opportunities for the members. Delegates from the state take state and/or member issues to the HOD for all members to have input into the functioning of the Academy.

Academy of Nutrition and Dietetics Foundation

The Academy of Nutrition and Dietetics Foundation is a nonprofit arm of the Academy that solicits and receives monies to benefit the Academy, with a large percentage of the monies going to provide scholarships for both undergraduate and graduate students and for member research projects. The foundation fosters alignment with corporate sponsors and conducts member campaigns for fund-raising. The foundation also provides services for the public in various ways.

More than 900 students have been awarded scholarships since 2007, totaling nearly $1.4 million. The Evidence Analysis Library, a resource offered through the Foundation, is a member-accessible online reference library housing relevant nutritional research on important dietetic practice questions. The service is also available through a subscription service to others.[13]

Washington Office

The Academy maintains an office in Washington, DC, to have a presence in the capital and further the legislative efforts of the profession. This allows the association to be in touch with legislative issues as they are being considered and as they occur. Although these legislative and lobbying efforts required a tax status change by the association when they were first initiated, the benefits accrue to individual members directly and to consumers and the public indirectly.

The staff of the Washington office and Academy members work with legislators and government agencies to introduce and promote bills that further the interests of the profession and its members. An example is the passage of the Medical Nutrition Therapy Act, which resulted from a sustained effort on the part of ADA staff together with legislators over several years. Members contribute to a political action committee (PAC) that makes awards to legislators who promote programs and activities important to the Academy.

American Overseas Dietetic Association

Dietitians who have met all requirements for membership in the Academy are eligible for membership in the overseas association. They may join DPGs and enjoy all the same benefits of membership as they would in the United States.

SUMMARY

The Academy of Nutrition and Dietetics is the professional organization serving and promoting the interests of its members. The programs and initiatives administered by the Academy are for the benefit of the members and the public. The Academy is governed by elected and appointed volunteer members of boards, commissions, and committees, all of whom perform specific functions according to the bylaws of the Academy. Important as the functions that the Academy provides for members are, it is recognized as the authoritative voice to the public with guidance regarding food and nutrition issues. The active promotion of policy that enhances the health and well-being of all individuals is accomplished through activities by members and by the Washington legislative office.

DEFINITIONS

Bylaws. Authoritative rules governing an association or group.

Chief executive officer (CEO). A person employed by the association to direct the headquarters office operations and implement the programs and fiscal affairs of the association. May also serve as an official spokesperson for the Academy on direction of the board of directors.

Governance. Activities involved in conducting the affairs of an organization.

Strategic plan. Plans and strategies that shape the overall activities and functions of an organization.

REFERENCES

1. Escott-Stump, S.A. "President's Page." *J Acad Nutr Diet* 112, no. 3 (2012): 352.
2. www.eatright.org (10/12/15).
3. Ibid.
4. Ibid.
5. Ibid.
6. Switt, J.T. "The American Dietetic Association's New Look." *J Am Diet Assoc* 108 (2008): 932–933.
7. Bylaws of the Academy of Nutrition and Dietetics. www.eatright.org (10/15/15)
8. Weinland, J., and L. Smothers. "2015 Academy Member Benefits Update." *J Acad Nutr Diet* 115, no. 4 (2015): 505–509.
9. Cassell, J. *Carry the Flame: The History of the American Dietetic Association.* (Chicago: The American Dietetic Association, 1990).
10. Baldyga, W.W. "Results from the 1981 Census of the American Dietetic Association." *J Am Diet Assoc* 83 (1983): 343–348.
11. Rogers, D. "Compensation and Benefits Survey 2015." *J Acad Nutr Diet* 116, no. 3 (2016): 370–388.
12. See Note 11.
13. Academy of Nutrition and Dietetics website. Accessed November 5, 2012, www.eatright.org

CHAPTER 3

Educational Preparation In Dietetics

"As a profession, the one thing that we can predict is that the greatest change in our practice will be the change in knowledge and how we integrate new science into our daily practice."[1]

OUTLINE

LEARNING OBJECTIVES

The student will be able to:
1. Discuss the academic requirements for practice in dietetics and membership in the Academy.
2. Compare the didactic program in dietetics and the coordinated program in dietetics.
3. Describe the standards of education and their purpose.
4. Understand the application process for supervised practice.
5. Understand how competencies for entry-level practice are integrated into supervised practice.
6. Know the basic requirements for advanced study and degrees.

INTRODUCTION

Education is the key to dietetic practice and to the future of the profession. As with all professionals, a specialized body of knowledge is required of individuals who practice in any area of dietetics. Because of the importance of education in the profession, early leaders in dietetics set standards for the education of dietitians. The standards have been revised at intervals as the practice evolved and the needs of those being served changed.

UNDERGRADUATE EDUCATION

The educational preparation of the dietitian begins in the undergraduate degree program. Study for the baccalaureate degree is based in the biological, physiological, behavioral, and social sciences, and it includes both theoretical and applied courses. The college or university offering a degree program plans a curriculum that meets both the educational standards of the Academy of Nutrition and Dietetics and the university requirements, including general education courses. A baccalaureate degree from an accredited college or university, combined with a supervised experience either integrated into the degree program or in an internship following the degree, is required to fulfill all education requirements.

A curriculum that meets the academic standards is referred to as a didactic program in dietetics (DPD). A program that offers the practical experience component concurrently with the degree is termed a coordinated program (CP). The dietetic technician (DT) program similarly follows a course of study in a 2-year college or institution that includes or is followed by a practice component.

DIETETICS EDUCATION PROGRAMS

Didactic Program in Dietetics

The didactic or classwork portion of the dietetics educational requirement is completed during the degree program, either undergraduate or graduate. Following the degree conferral, the student completes a supervised practice program or internship. The traditional didactic program is a 4-year bachelor of science degree. Many of the courses required in the DPD combine classroom and laboratory work, especially in food production, clinical nutrition, and science courses such as chemistry and microbiology.

During the latter part of the program, usually the senior year, the student applies to one or more dietetic internships through a computerized matching program. Notification is given in April or November about a match or acceptance to the student's program of choice. After completion of the supervised portion of the program, the student may take the registration examination.

Coordinated Program in Dietetics

In the coordinated program (CP) in dietetics, the didactic portion of a program and supervised practice are completed during the course of study toward the degree, either undergraduate or graduate. The student graduating from this program is prepared for entry-level practice upon completion of the degree. In most universities, students enter the CP for their junior and senior years. The program is sometimes described as a "two-by-two," meaning the first 2 years are general study and may be at a community or junior college and the last 2 include the integrated courses leading to the degree. Some programs may be longer than the traditional 4 years, depending on the specific program requirements.

A university designates the criteria for admission to the CP. The selection criteria commonly include grade point average, writing skill, work experience, letters of recommendation, and, sometimes, an interview. A minimum of 1200 hours of supervised practice is required in the CP. The program is intense in terms of time requirements and experiences but can reduce the time needed to prepare for practice. On completion of the degree, the student is eligible to take the registration examination.

Dietetic Technician Program

The dietetic technician (DT) program is similar to the CP in that both didactic and supervised practice (minimum of 450 clock hours) are required. The Accreditation Council for Education in Nutrition and Dietetics (ACEND) also accredits the programs. Graduates of the program may also become registered by taking the DTR examination. Many of the programs are offered in 2-year colleges or technical schools.

EDUCATION PROGRAM STANDARDS

ACEND sets the standards by which dietitians are educated. The standards have been issued in various forms since 1924 and have undergone many changes in both concept and form. For instance, early emphasis was on the specific courses a student was required to take during a degree program. Now, the standards are based on the outcomes expected from the education experience, and education program directors translate the expected outcomes into courses and course content. ACEND further specifies how a degree program is structured, including the goals and philosophy of the program, the students, the curriculum, the program resources, and evaluation of the program.

The standards for all degree and experience program include the following:[2]

1. Program characteristics and resources
2. Mission, goals, and objectives of the program
3. Curriculum learning activities
4. Faculty and preceptors
5. Supervised practice and learning sites
6. Information for prospective students and the public
7. Policies and procedures
8. Program evaluation and improvement

The ACEND evaluates each educational program through an accreditation site visit based on an extensive self-study prepared by the program director and staff. The purpose of the site visit, conducted by registered dietitians designated by ACEND, is to assist the program in continued assessment that ensures qualified, competent program graduates who pass the registration examination and are prepared to practice. A program may be accredited for a period of 5 to 10 years. Periodic reports are submitted to the Academy indicating that the program continues to provide education that meets the standards. A list of all accredited programs is available from a college or university or from the Academy website.

SUPERVISED PRACTICE IN DIETETICS

Preprofessional or supervised practice is an essential step toward becoming a registered dietitian nutritionist (RDN) or nutrition and dietetics technician, registered (NDTR). For the DPD student, the dietetic internship follows the degree. Supervised practice takes place in the work setting where students learn to apply their knowledge and skills under the direction of a preceptor. Successful completion of supervised practice program establishes eligibility for an individual to take the registration examination and apply for active membership in the Academy. Competency in dietetics practice is the goal of supervised practice. Competency is regarded as the ability to carry out tasks within certain expected standards or parameters.

Supervised practice programs are based on the standards of education and the competencies for entry-level practice. All supervised programs must offer a minimum of 1200 hours of experience for the dietitian and 450 hours for the DT. A current listing of all programs is available on the Academy website.

Programs follow the same standards; however, there is flexibility in the way the programs meet the standards through the kinds of experiences offered. Although ACEND accredits the educational programs, it does not mandate the kinds of experiences or the amount of time in each area of practice. Each program sets the curriculum and experiences that meet the goals of the program and the needs of the student.

Experiences are structured around three key areas of activity in dietetics: clinical nutrition, food service management, and community dietetics. Programs that do not offer all the experiences in one institution will arrange with others in the community or area to provide them.

Besides the dietetic internship, the CP, and the DT practice, the Individualized Supervised Practice Pathway (ISSP) also offers a pathway to registration and membership.[3] The ISSP, offered in 2015 in 11 programs, provides a way for persons not matched for an internship placement to gain experience and for doctoral students not holding a verification statement or having completed didactic course work. Requirements for acceptance to the program are determined by the institution or program offering the experience as is the choice of a preceptor for the student.

What do students need to know before applying to a supervised experience program? Students should know that a period of supervised experience is required to establish eligibility to become an RDN or NDTR and that acceptance into a program is competitive. The application process should begin early in the senior year to assemble all required materials by graduation and, if required by the program desired by the student, to visit one or more programs. Students applying for a dietetic internship will usually participate in the national computer matching. Information about this process may be obtained from the program director or the Academy.

What are the characteristics of successful applicants? Generally, applicants with a grade point average of 3.0 or above in food, nutrition, and management courses and better than average in biological and physical science courses will be considered first. Approximately 1 year of work experience or dietetics-related volunteer or paid experience will increase the chance of being chosen.

What else is important to know? In addition to good grades and work experience, applicants are encouraged to investigate programs early to identify the specific admission criteria and to apply to one or more. Successful applicants often apply to as many as three programs. If the program requires or offers graduate credit during the supervised experience, the student will need to apply to graduate school and complete the graduate record examination (GRE). In addition, applicants are encouraged to be flexible and be willing to relocate if necessary.

Program directors who advise students and students themselves need to have other options in mind when an internship appointment is not obtained. Some plan to gain more working experience and then reapply. Another alternative is an advanced degree. Some students gain additional training or complete course work for allied health areas such as nursing, physician assistant, or physical therapy. Employment areas that in most cases do not require the RD credential might also be considered. Examples are pharmaceutical companies, journalism and communications, hospitality, athletic training spas and centers, tourism, retirement homes, cooperative extension, and school food service.

ADVANCED-LEVEL EDUCATION

Advanced-level education may be described as continuing education, pre-professional education, or graduate education. More baccalaureate students are pursuing a graduate degree; more employers are requiring an advanced degree, training, or advanced credentials; and more disciplines are becoming specialized, thus requiring advanced-level education. Graduate education is formal study beyond a baccalaureate degree that leads to an advanced degree, that is, the master's or doctoral degree. Graduate study involves concentrated work in a specific academic area. Some universities offer or require graduate study concurrently with the dietetic internship.

Among the purposes of advanced education are opportunities for individuals to explore new ideas and gain a higher level of knowledge and understanding required to recognize and fully discharge personal, social, and professional responsibilities. Practical benefits also accrue, including networking with other advanced practitioners and specialists, the possibility of career advancement and financial gain.

Types of Programs

The master of science (MS) degree usually requires 1 to 2 years of full-time study and may be longer depending on the major area of study, the research undertaken, and whether the student attends full or part-time. The doctor of philosophy (PhD) or doctor of education (EdD) usually requires a minimum of 3 years of full-time study. Original research and a thesis or dissertation, or an equivalent academic work, will be required depending on the field of study and the requirements of the educational institution. The doctoral degree is considered the terminal degree although, at times, it will be followed by postdoctoral academic study.

Some allied healthcare disciplines offer a "practice doctorate" for advanced-level degree study. This has also been proposed in dietetics by Academy members and may be a consideration in the future as another route to advanced work.[4]

Benefits of Advanced Study

The benefits of an advanced degree include the development of intellectual skills such as the ability to master complex information, problem solve, and explore new ideas. Career benefits include the development of advanced practice skills, the in-depth exploration of subjects in one's area of practice or in another area, and the acquisition of new perspectives. Dietitians often pursue graduate study for career advancement or preparation for a career change. Dietitians who are prepared to perform in multiskilled or cross-trained positions will usually rely on graduate education to increase their knowledge and practice skills.

The type of positions dietitians assume as they progress in their careers are usually those with increasing responsibility and autonomy that require management and leadership skills. Competition for jobs may also increase the demand for advanced degrees. New and expanding career options and the job market in general affects demand and availability and, in turn, may influence dietitians in their education choices. Graduate education provides an opportunity to develop expertise that allows dietitians to assume leadership roles.

In the 2015 Compensation and Benefits survey, it was reported that over half (52 percent) of RDNs hold an advanced degree. Among NDTRs, 57 percent hold the Associate degree and 39 percent the bachelor's degree.[5]

The financial advantage of an advanced degree for RDNs is shown in **Table 3-1**. The dietitian with a master's degree receives $500 more and the doctoral degree $30,000 more than a person with the bachelor's

Table 3-1. Median Yearly Income of Registered Dietitians by Education Level

Degree Level	2011[a]	2013[b]	2015[c]
Bachelor degree	55,000	57,574	60,008
Master degree	60,000	61,506	65,478
Doctoral degree	75,000	75,005	92,000
ALL RDs	58,000	60,000	63,700

Sources: a. Ward, B. "Compensation and Benefits Survey 2011: Moderate Growth in Registered Dietitian and Dietetic Technician, Registered, Compensation in the past 2 years." *J Acad Nutr Diet* 112, no. 1 (2012): 29–40.

b. Rogers, D. "Compensation and Benefits Survey 2013; Education and Job Responsibility Key to Increased Compensation." *J Acad Nutr Diet* 114, no. 1 (2014): 17–33.

c. Rogers, D. "Compensation and Benefits Survey 2015." *J Acad Diet* 116, no. 3 (2016): 370–388.

degree. State licensure and specialty certification affect salaries and are often equated with advanced study. Dietitians working in practice areas that often require an advanced degree, such as food and nutrition management and education and research, earn the highest salaries. For NDTRs, the median yearly wage is $42,000—an increase from $40,000 in 2013. The factors affecting salaries are about the same as for the NRD—education, experience, responsibility, and location. The NDTRs in food and nutrition management generally earn the highest salaries.

Other reasons to pursue graduate study are for continuing education credit to maintain registration status, when state licensure regulations mandate an advanced degree and continuing education, and for gaining research skills and understanding research reports. All dietitians apply research in their practice and need to demonstrate the ability to interpret current research and basic statistics.

The Graduate Program Experience

Information about graduate programs is available in the Academy Directory of Programs and from universities. Prospective students find it helpful to talk with faculty and to request college catalogs and departmental information before applying. No two programs are alike and the best fit between the student and the program will be important once the student is admitted. Universities that give the student an active role in departmental activities as well as individual time in a mentoring and supporting atmosphere will greatly enhance the graduate experience. Departmental research and the availability of financial aid should also be explored. Assistantships give financial aid and teaching, research, and/or administrative experiences according to assignments.

Research Experience

The selection of a research study is based on an area of interest, the need as determined by a literature search, and the feasibility of the study (based on cost, time involvement, and availability of equipment and/or subjects). Ongoing departmental research by faculty can provide a way for the student to assume a part of the research.

The process of investigating a problem, reviewing the literature, planning and implementing the study, collecting and analyzing data, and writing a clear and well-developed document that is accepted by a graduate faculty committee is a significant effort. The research experience requires initiative, critical thinking, problem solving, and ethical procedures. The successful completion of a research study often launches a student into publishing the results and into further research, thus making an important contribution to scholarship.

DISTANCE EDUCATION

Distance education is the means by which many colleges and universities now offer courses and degree programs. With the increased use of technology by both students and practitioners, such offerings are often attractive to part-time students, older returning students, and others who reside away from a university setting. Three universities now offer the DPD by distance. In 2015, 26 internships also offered part of the curriculum by distance.[6]

An example of an established, successful distance education program is the Great Plains Interactive Distance Education Alliance (IDEA) that offers the master's degree. The alliance is composed of 12 universities in the Midwest who offer a common core of subjects with elective options offered by the individual universities. The degree is granted by the university in which the student is enrolled.[7]

"A Guide for Effective Nutrition Intervention and Education" (GENIE) is an online resource for the assessment of the quality of a program.[8] By using a checklist of nine categories, a program director can determine how effective a program is and make any necessary adjustments.

A large-scale online distance opportunity is available through the "Massive Open Online Courses" (MOOCS).[9] Free courses are open to anyone worldwide. Enrollments of several thousand are not unusual as evidenced by a course offered by Cornell University on "Infant and Young Child Feeding" with thousands enrolled. A variety of instructional methods are used along with tests.

Continuing education opportunities for professionals are increasingly offered by distance through webinars, teleconferences, teleseminars, and social networking means. The annual public policy workshop is now offered by distance. Many dietetic practice groups regularly communicate through blogs, Facebook, Twitter, and Skype.

In some locations, patient health care is provided through a "telehealth" system. Medical nutrition therapy may be a part of the practice as well as consultation in business and private practice. Legal and ethical considerations as well as professionalism are important when these means of communication are used.[10]

FUTURE EDUCATION PREPARATION

The education of the dietitian focuses on the present and future roles professionals will fulfill. The traditional roles continue to expand as environmental, demographic business, and health trends create new opportunities for practice. ACEND, working with the Council on Future Practice, plans toward future practice and education needs. In 2013, they initiated an Environmental Scan that revealed emerging nontraditional practice settings for nutrition and dietetics and an expanding scope of practice in the profession. For instance, there is an increased focus on disease prevention and integrative health care. There is also a need for more knowledge in areas such as nutritional pharmacology, case management, behavioral counseling, prescriptive authority, coding and reimbursement, evidence-based practice, and informatics. There is also a growing importance for healthcare professionals to work more interprofessionally.

As an outcome of the environmental scan, ACEND made several recommendations:[11]

1. The requirement of a minimum of the master's degree as preparation for an entry-level, generalist, registered dietitian nutritionist.
2. The bachelor's degree required for entry-level nutrition and dietetics technician.
3. Associate degree preparation for nutrition health workers.
4. Competencies to be identified for each degree level.
5. Experiential learning integrated into each degree program.
6. Each degree level prepares students for employment.
7. Future exploration of high school and doctoral level programs.

Some of the recommendations have been approved and others are under study for their implications for the future of education and practice. One that has been approved is the requirement for the master's degree for the entry-level RDN will be implemented as of 2024.[12] Another is supervised practice integrated into the didactic program.

New standards for all degree and experience programs were developed by ACEND in 2016 to be implemented upon finalization in 2017.[13]

SUMMARY

Dietetics education has evolved over time but has always been based on preparing the student for professional practice. The Academy designates the educational standards that are followed by all dietetics programs, thus ensuring competent practitioners. With a background of academic knowledge and practical skills, dietitians and DTs are prepared for a wide variety of careers.

Over half of practicing dietitians today hold a graduate degree. There are benefits in doing so—research competence, continuing education for personal and professional growth, and career enhancement. Even more dietitians will receive advanced education as the new education requirements become effective. The outcome will be an informed public and a heightened recognition of the dietitian as the expert in food and nutrition and a member of interprofessional teams.

DEFINITIONS

Accreditation. The process whereby a private nongovernmental agency or association grants public recognition to an institution or an individual who meets necessary qualifications and periodic evaluation.

Advanced study. Study beyond the traditional baccalaureate level.

Advanced practice. Effective discharge of job requirements that demonstrates a high level of skills, knowledge, and behaviors.

Coordinated program (CP). A degree undergraduate program that combines didactic and experiential learning.

Preceptor. A person who guides, mentors, and evaluates a student during supervised practice.

Specialist. One who possesses a proficient level of knowledge, skill, and experience to qualify for a specific credential.

Supervised practice. Learning experiences associated with activities guided by a leader or preceptor.

REFERENCES

1. Parks, S.D., M.R. Schiller, and J. Bryk. "President's Page." *J Am Diet Assoc* 12 (1994): 1159–1161.

2. 2017 Education Program Standards. Accreditation Council for Education and Dietetics. www.eatright.org/ACEND

3. Wilson, A. New Supervised Practice Pathway Offers Additional Options to Dietetics Graduate. ADA Times 9, no. 1 (2011): 18–19.

4. Skipper, A., and N.M., Lewis. "Clinical Registered Dietitians, Employers, and Educators are Interested in Advanced Practice Education and Professional Doctorate Degrees in Clinical Nutrition." *J Am Diet Assoc* 106, no. 12 (2006): 2062–2066.

5. Rogers, D. "Compensation and Benefits Survey 2015." *J Acad Nutr Diet* 116, no. 3 (2016): 370–388.

6. www.eatright.org

7. http://www.gpidea.org/

8. www.eatright.PRO.org/GENIE.

9. Stark, C.M. "Massive Open Online Courses: How Registered Dietitians Use MOOCS for Nutrition Education." *J Acad Nutr Diet* 114, no. 8 (2014): 1147–1155.

10. Ayres, E.J. "The Impact of Social Media and Business and Ethical Practices in Dietetics." *J Acad Nutr Diet* 113, no. 11 (2013): 1539–1543.

11. Rationale for Future Education Preparation of Nutrition and Dietetics Practitioners. www.eatright.org/ACEND. August 2015.

12. www.eatright.org/ACEND. August 2016.

13. See Note 2.

CHAPTER 4

Credentialing of Nutrition and Dietetic Practitioners

"Nutrition and dietetics credentialing protects and improves the health of the public and supports practitioner competence, quality practice, lifelong learning and career advancement."
Vision Statement of The Commission on Dietetic Registration[1]

OUTLINE

- Learning Objectives
- Introduction
- Development of Credentialing
- Commission on Dietetic Registration
- Registered Dietitian Nutritionist
- Dietetic Technician, Registered or Nutrition and Dietetics Technician, Registered
- New Dietetic Technician Registration Elgibility Pathway
  - Examination Candidate Information and Study Resources
- Specialist Certification
- Interdisciplinary Specialist Certification in Obesity and Weight Management
- Advanced Practice Certification in Clinical Nutrition
- Certificates of Training
- Recertification of the RD/RDN and DTR/NDTR

- Recertification of Specialists and Advanced Practice in Clinical Nutrition
- Appropriate Use of Credentials
- Legal Regulation Statutes for Dietitians Nutritionists and Dietetic Technicians
- Summary
- Definitions
- References

LEARNING OBJECTIVES

The student will be able to:

1. Understand the importance of credentialing for practice.
2. Become familiar with the Commission on Dietetic Registration and how it functions.
3. Know the academic and test requirements for becoming credentialed.
4. Become familiar with the certification and recertification process and the portfolio requirements.
5. Become aware of the requirements for specialization in dietetics.
6. Know the legal requirements pertaining to certification of dietitians and nutritionists.

INTRODUCTION

The term *dietitian* is one that evolved over time. Early practitioners were called dietologists, dietists, and dietotherapists.[2] Before the American Dietetic Association (ADA) was formed, (currently the Academy of Nutrition and Dietetics), a dietitian was described as "a person who specializes in the knowledge of food and can meet the demands of the medical profession for diet therapy."[3] This adequately described the professional for many decades. Today the Academy defines a dietitian: "A dietitian is a person who is trained in the science of nutrition and dietetics."[4]

The science of food and nutrition formed the basis for the organization of a group of practicing professionals. One of the earliest concerns of this group was the overwhelming amount of food faddism and fallacies found among the general public and even among other professionals. It was difficult, if not impossible, for the public to determine who was a credible source of information and to separate fact from fiction between the many medical and health claims for specific foods and procedures.

This early concern for protection of the public by disseminating the knowledge of dietitians has continued to the present time. Not only did it lead to the national organization of dietitians that could promote the professionals as having expertise in "diet-therapy, teaching, social welfare, and administration," but it served as the impetus to begin thinking about credentialing of practitioners.

A concern raised at the second annual meeting of the ADA in 1918 was the "need to distinguish between dietitians with a college degree and special training in some scientific work and the ones with lesser training."[5]

This was perhaps the first formal reference to dietetic credentialing. The 1926 president of the association, Florence Smith, urged that the group establish professional standards for dietitians and that state or national registration could be the answer. In 1929, a study of national registration was initiated, and the following definition of a dietitian was adopted: "Any person who is qualified for membership in The American Dietetic Association is by virtue of uniform basic training and required experience, entitled to be designated as a dietitian."[6] In the 1950s, the association appointed a committee to formally study state licensure of dietitians.[7] The issue of specialties in practice also surfaced with the suggestion that membership should be expanded to include others who were well qualified in the many specialties embraced within the definition of dietetics.[8] Although certification of dietitians occurred in the late 1960s, it was not until the late 1990s that education and membership requirements were differentiated to accommodate practitioners with similar basic preparation but in specialized or focused areas of practice.

The differences between a generalist and a specialist surfaced and were thoroughly debated. A generalist was defined as a dietitian who could perform in all areas of practice, such as a single dietitian in a small hospital, or one who could move from one practice area to another. A specialist was a dietitian wanting to restrict his or her practice in one area, such as clinical or food service. The generalist role was advanced by the following themes:

1. All dietitians are the same.
2. Dietitians can move from one area of practice to another (food service to public health, for example) without additional training.
3. Greater external recognition of the term *dietitian* was established.

By contrast, the specialized role was driven by the following themes:

1. The explosion of knowledge and technology required each dietitian to know more and more about less and less.
2. There was a need to differentiate among dietitians with varying skills and knowledge, advanced education, and experience gained on the job.
3. Part-time employment opportunities emerged.
4. New, innovative practice areas developed, such as school food service, nursing home consultation, enteral and parenteral nutrition techniques, and nutrition support.

DEVELOPMENT OF CREDENTIALING

In the 1960s, a committee was established to study licensure, registration, and certification. Registration was the credentialing process chosen at that time by the ADA House of Delegates and the ADA membership. An amendment to the constitution was approved for the *Final Revised Proposal for Professional Registration* in 1969.[9] A committee, later to become known as the Commission on Dietetic Registration (CDR), then began the implementation of a certification process for members. The title for those ADA members who chose to become certified was registered dietitian (RD). A detailed account of the implementation and a review of the first 5 years of professional registration were published in the *Journal of the American Dietetic Association* in 1974.[10]

The professional registration system adopted by the association differed significantly from other health professional certification systems at that time in that candidates had to pass a national examination, and RDs had to document evidence of continuing education in each 5-year period to renew registration. Thus registration was designed as a voluntary process to ensure competency of dietitians through the qualifications required to take the registration examination, passing the examination, and formal continuing education. All of this was evidence of the concern of the profession for the health, safety, and welfare of the public by encouraging high standards of performance by dietetic practitioners as stated in the amendment to the constitution.

By late 1970, 90 percent of the membership was registered, with the majority grandfathered in during the period before establishment of the examination. Credentialing of the dietetic technician and various dietetic specialists followed with qualifications developed by the Commission on Dietetic Registration.[11]

COMMISSION ON DIETETIC REGISTRATION

The mission of the Commission on Dietetic Registration (CDR), as the credentialing agency and organization unit of the Academy of Nutrition and Dietetics (AND, referred to as the Academy), is to administer rigorous, valid, and reliable credentialing processes to protect the public and meet the needs of CDR's credentialed practitioners, employers, and consumers.

Credentialed practitioners elect the Commission members for 3-year terms. Members of the Commission elect the CDR Chair.

The Commission's RDN, RD, NDTR, and DTR certification programs are fully accredited by the National Commission for Certifying Agencies (NCCA), the accrediting arm of the Institute for Credentialing Excellence based in Washington, DC. This accreditation reflects achievement of the highest standards of professional credentialing. As of early 2016, CDR was maintaining a registry of more than 100,000 dietetic practitioners. CDR is the administratively autonomous credentialing agency for the Academy and develops, revises, and administers the examination for registration; sets the standards for certification and recertification; establishes the Code of Ethics for the Profession of Dietetics jointly with the Academy; and issues credentials to individuals who meet these standards for competency to practice in the dietetics profession.[12,13]

REGISTERED DIETITIAN NUTRITIONIST

CDR establishes the requirements for eligibility to take the entry-level examination for dietitians. Requirements include academic preparation, supervised practice, and confirmation of academic and practice requirements by online verification. The examination is administered online and individual applicants can schedule a time to take it throughout the year. The examination is also available in other countries from organizations with which the Academy has reciprocity. Currently those are Dietitians of Canada, the Dutch Association of Dietitians, the Philippine Professional Regulation Commission, and the Irish Nutrition and Dietetic Institute. Traditionally the academic eligibility requirements to take the registered dietitian nutritionist (RDN/RD) examination was the completion of a baccalaureate degree from a U.S. regionally accredited college or university or foreign equivalent.

The Council on Future Practice Visioning Report of 2012 recommended changing the requirement from a baccalaureate degree to a minimum of a graduate degree. The full report is now available.[14] That formed the basis for CDR to change the entry-level education requirements for dietitians beginning January 1, 2024, from a baccalaureate degree to a minimum of a graduate degree.

Detailed explanation of all of the current eligibility requirements may be accessed at: http:www.cdrnet.org. They are subject to change and the most reliable information is on the CDR website. Additional details of the academic requirements can be accessed at: http://www.eatrightacend.org.

After passing the examination and being credentialed by CDR, registered dietitians (RD and RDN) are required to comply with CDR recertification requirements, the "Code of Ethics for the Profession of Dietetics," the "Scope of Practice for the Registered Dietitian," and the "Revised 2012 Standards of Practice in Nutrition Care and Standards of Professional Performance for Registered Dietitians."[15–17]

DIETETIC TECHNICIAN, REGISTERED OR NUTRITION AND DIETETICS TECHNICIAN, REGISTERED

CDR establishes the eligibility requirements for dietetic technicians. Currently the requirement is completion of an Associate degree granted by a regionally accredited college or university with the Accreditation Council for Education in Nutrition and Dietetics (ACEND) accredited Dietetic Technician Program. http://eatrightacend.org.

The dietetic technician, registered (DTR) or nutrition and dietetics technician, registered (NDTR) is a critical member of the dietetics team and has become even more important as the practice of dietetics in every area becomes more complicated and time consuming and with the increasing number of opportunities for employment. Dietetic technicians are trained in food and nutrition and are an integral part of health care, food service, and other dietetics and healthcare teams. In small, rural hospitals, the DTR/NDTR is sometimes the only trained dietetics practitioner addressing all aspects of care available full time. In this situation, the DTR/NDTR works under the supervision of an RD/RDN via established protocols to implement the nutrition care process based on state regulations. The "Scope of Dietetic Practice for the Dietetic Technician, Registered" published in 2013 addresses supervision, entry-level, and advanced practice for DTRs.[18]

Currently the small number of DTRs and dietetic technician educational programs place this segment of our profession at risk for continued existence. An increase in the number of DTRs/NDTRs is vital to sustain expansion of practice areas for dietitians and achieve the future vision for the profession.

A functional career ladder for dietetic technicians discussed below as a new pathway for technicians will strengthen the dietetics profession as we seek to enhance the recognition, authority, autonomy, prestige, income, and satisfaction of dietetics team members and their customers.

It is well known that NDTR/DTRs work in nontraditional or emerging areas of practice with more diverse possibilities for the future. After appropriate years of practice, NDTR/DTRs also may work with RDN/RDs in advanced-level practice. The use of the "Scope of Practice for the Dietetic Technician, Registered" and the "Revised 2012 Standards of Practice in Nutrition Care and Standards of Professional Performance for Dietetic Technicians, Registered" addresses this issue of advanced practice for DTRs.[19,20]

The opportunities for employment keep expanding for the DTR, especially in areas where supply of RDN/RDs cannot meet the demand. More and more employers, especially in the healthcare arena, are requiring that an individual be credentialed as a DTR/NDTR in order to practice in their facilities. Some current unique opportunities are:

- Supervising food safety and sanitation in a variety of public and private venues

- Assisting individuals and groups in wellness and fitness centers to know how food relates to fitness
- Managing and directing food service employees in assisted living and retirement centers
- Assisting the RD/RDN in collecting data from patients or participants in research studies (in hospitals, clinics, and community research centers)

The *Final Report of the Phase 2 Future Practice and Education Task Force* provides more detail of innovative educational experiences and unique roles and employment for DTRs both now and in the future.[21]

In summary, the DTR/NDTR of today will extend the scope of practice for the RD/RDN in the future and will allow the RD/RDNs to delegate responsibilities, enabling them to practice at specialty and advanced levels. However, for this to happen, the RD/RDN must understand the role and appropriate responsibilities of the DTR/NDTR, which will increase visibility and credibility of the dietetic professional team and benefit clients, facilities, and the profession of dietetics. Last but not least, dietetic professionals and the Academy must promote the value of DTR/NDTR educational programs and the dietetic technician as a creditable member of the team for practice in tomorrow's world.

NEW DIETETIC TECHNICIAN REGISTRATION ELIGIBILITY PATHWAY

For the past several years, the CDR and others have noted the decline in the number of technicians. This decline has been complicated by the lack of educational programs for technicians in many states, resulting in employers being unable to find appropriately trained technicians and increasing the unavailability of technicians in the United States.

The CDR has supported the role of the technician and believes that a new pathway will address both of these issues. This decision is consistent with the CDR's public protection mission in that it provides a credential for the numerous non-credentialed Didactic Programs in Dietetics (DPD) graduates currently employed in dietetic technician positions. Once credentialed as DTR/NDTRs, these individuals will be required to comply with the CDR recertification requirements. The CDR also believes that this alternative registration eligibility option will provide a dietetics career ladder, increase the availability and visibility of DTR/NDTRs throughout the country, and ultimately enhance the value of the DTR/NDTR credential.[22] The *Dietetics Career Development Guide* uses the Dreyfus model of skill acquisition to show how practitioners can attain increasing levels of knowledge and skills throughout a career.[23,24]

In 2009, CDR established a New Pathway III for dietetic technicians. Individuals who complete both a baccalaureate degree and a DPD will be able to take the registration examination for dietetic technicians without meeting additional academic or supervised practice requirements. This decision also provides for the numerous non-credentialed DPD graduates currently employed in dietetic technician positions to become credentialed. The CDR also believes that this alternative registration eligibility option will increase the availability and visibility of DTRs throughout the country, ultimately enhancing the value of the DTR credential.

Effective June 1, 2009, the two pathways to establish eligibility to take the registration examinations for dietetic technicians are:

1. *Pathway I.* Completion of an associate's degree granted by a U.S. regionally accredited college or university with the Accreditation Council for Education in Nutrition and Dietetics (ACEND) Accredited Dietetic Technician Program.
2. *Pathway III.* Completion of a baccalaureate degree granted by a U.S. regionally accredited college or university, or foreign equivalent, completion of an ACEND-accredited Didactic Program in Dietetics (DPD), and completion of an ACEND-accredited dietetic technician supervised practice.

All dietetic technician Pathway III candidates must be submitted for registration eligibility by their graduating institution's current DPD director. In addition, candidates must complete an electronic application available on the CDR's website at: https://www.cdrnet.org.

After passing the registration examination for dietetic technicians and being credentialed by the CDR, DTRs/NDTRs are required to comply with CDR recertification requirements, the "Code of Ethics for the Profession of Dietetics," "Scope of Practice for the Dietetic Technician, Registered and the Revised 2012 Standards of Practice in Nutrition Care and Standards of Professional Performance for Dietetic Technicians, Registered."[25–27]

The following are additional Academy and CDR webpages of importance to individuals preparing for certification as dietetic technicians:

Examination Candidate Information and Study Resources

Computer-based testing FAQ:

> https://www.cdrnet.org/vault/2459/web/files/CBTFactSheet082015
> .pdf
> *Study Guide for the Registration Examination for Dietetic Technicians*, 6th ed. https://www.eatrightstore.org/product
> /2ACAE4B2-2092-46D5-9435-0710C45CC866

SPECIALIST CERTIFICATION

The concept of specialized practice in dietetics was approved by the ADA House of Delegates in 1986. Currently, the Academy defines a specialist as a practitioner who demonstrates additional knowledge, skills, and experience in a focus area of dietetics practice by the attainment of a credential.[28] Three areas of practice were selected for initial certification: pediatric nutrition, renal nutrition, and metabolic nutrition care. The metabolic nutrition care specialist was later discontinued.

New criteria were established for the specialist, which include education and experience requirements as well as the successful completion of the CDR examination in the focus area. Specialists are currently credentialed in the following areas:

Gerontological Nutrition
Sports Dietetics
Pediatric Nutrition
Renal Nutrition
Oncology Nutrition

As of 2016, one additional specialty certification will be available: Board Certified Specialist in Obesity and Weight Management (Interdisciplinary Certification). This is the first certificate offered as an "interdisciplinary" certificate. Additional information about this specialist certification is presented later in this chapter.

Although minimum eligibility requirements (Current RD/DRN status with CDR, passing an examination in the focus area, maintenance of

RD/RDN status with CDR, and documentation of practice experience) for the specialists listed above are similar, there are some differences in specifics. Therefore, it is necessary for candidates to access the CDR website (https://www.cdrnet.org) for current information on certification and recertification in a specific focus area.

INTERDISCIPLINARY SPECIALIST CERTIFICATION IN OBESITY AND WEIGHT MANAGEMENT

In 2013 the Council of Future Practice was (the Academy unit charged with the evaluation of new specialist certification petitions) presented with a petition from the Weight Management (WMDPG) and the Diabetes Care and Education (DCEDPG) practice groups for the development of a new obesity and weight management certification for Registered Dietitian Nutritionists (RDN). In July 2013, CDR agreed to move forward on the recommendation of the Future Council of Practice to proceed with the new specialist certification. Later in the year representatives of the petitioning groups (WMDPG and DCEDPG) along with representatives from the Obesity Society asked CDR to consider offering this certificate as an "interdisciplinary" certification. CDR appointed a Task Force that included representatives from the Academy Board of Directors, Council of Future Practice, Weight Management and Diabetes Care, and Education DPGs to consider this recommendation. After receiving comments from Academy membership and further discussion, CDR indicated that pros and cons received were evenly split. After much deliberation CDR agreed to move forward with the development process. The Task Force recommended that other allied health professionals be invited to participate in the practice audit: nurse practitioners, physician assistants, licensed clinical psychologists, clinical exercise physiologists, and licensed clinical social workers be included. In drafting the practice analysis survey instrument additional practitioners involved in weight management and representatives from the American College of Sports Medicine (ACSM), its Health Fitness Specialist, and Society of Behavioral Medicine (SBM), its Licensed Professional Counselor, and Licensed Marriage and Family Therapist were included. After the audit is complete, the professionals to be included for potential certification will be known. CDR has projected that the first examination for the specialist certification will be administered in the fall of 2016.

Raynor and Champagne provide further background information of the role of the dietitian in the weight management area.[29] They discuss the development of the position of the Academy as to interventions and treatment of overweight and obesity in adults.

Additional information about the process, practice audit results, and minimum eligibility, maintenance and documentation of experience requirements for the interdisciplinary board certified specialist is available at: https://www.cdrnet.org/weight-management. Professionals certified will be known as Board Certified Specialist in Obesity and Weight Management (CSOWM).

ADVANCED PRACTICE CERTIFICATION IN CLINICAL NUTRITION

Practitioners continued to pursue avenues to distinguish between entry level and advanced levels of practice.[30] An additional recognition was developed in 1993 for those practicing at advanced levels in any area of dietetics. Individual professionals were designated as: Fellow of the American Dietetic Association (FADA). This certification was available until 2003 for those having an advanced degree, 8 years of practice, plus other documented professional achievements. This FADA recognition was discontinued because of limited participation of members of the Academy. See Chapter 2 for details of a new fellows program (Fellow of Academy of Nutrition and Dietetics [FAND]) under membership benefits of the Academy.

Research and discussion within the Academy continued to address the issue of career ladders and levels of practice, including advanced practice.[31,32] Future roles and definitions for RD/RDNs, DTR/Ns, specialists, and advanced practice were further delineated in 2011 by the Council on Future Practice.[33]

CDR conducted a practice audit from 2005 to 2007 to identify and delineate advanced levels of practice (ALP) in nutrition and dietetics with the goal of determining the need for an advanced level of practice credential.[34] This study suggested that focus areas in clinical nutrition, community nutrition, management, business, and education/research were identified as having some unique ALP characteristics and needing further study. Other papers have shown the effort of numerous practitioners in moving this effort forward.[35–39]

The focus area of clinical nutrition was chosen as the initial area for an audit study and to develop, if feasible, an ALP credential. This seemed appropriate as clinical nutrition represents the largest practice group of practitioners in the Academy. In 2013 CDR appointed the Advanced Level Clinical Practice Audit Task Force.[40]

A subsequent article, "Developing an Advanced Practice Credential for Registered Dietitian Nutritionists in Clinical Practice," authored by Brody et al, provides details of the proceedings necessary to design and develop a new certification program for practitioners in advanced clinical nutrition practice as identified by the 2013 practice audit.[41]

CDR has described the profile of practitioners achieving the ALP credential in clinical dietetics as "experienced registered dietitians who have the knowledge and skills required to autonomously apply the nutrition care process at an optimal level of accuracy and efficiency" (http://www .cdrnet.org). The initial deadline for eligibility applications was set for August 6, 2016. Examinations are scheduled for November 2016 with the anticipation that a new group of registered dietitians would achieve the credential of Advanced Practice Certification in Clinical Nutrition (RDN-AP or RD_AP) in late 2016.

CERTIFICATES OF TRAINING

As the epidemic of obesity continues and the need for registered dietitians to become more involved in the efforts to prevent and treat obesity, the CDR offers three certificates of training in weight management. These certificates are in Childhood and Adolescent Weight Management, Adult Weight Management, and a Level 2 Certificate in Adult Weight Management. The certificate programs are designed to develop practitioners of comprehensive weight management care for adults, children, and adolescents. The certificates are available only for active, student, international and retired members of the Academy, and CDR credentialed practitioners: RDN, RD, NDTR, and DTR. As of mid-2015 over 20,000 practitioners have received a certificate with the majority from the adult weight management area.

Training for the certificates includes:

- State-of-the-art information and skills shared by leading practitioners
- Hands-on experience with cases and exercises

- Reference and other resource materials
- A range of 32 to 50 continuing professional education units (CPEUs) depending on the individual certificates

This training and the subsequent certificates have become very useful and popular with dietetic professionals returning to the workplace, working in private practice, and to registered dietitians in general. There is no reissue of the certificates, but certificate holders are encouraged to participate in retraining as needed. Additional information can be found at the CDR website: https://www.cdrnet.org/weight-management.

RECERTIFICATION OF THE RD/RDN AND DTR/NDTR

In 2001, the CDR implemented a new process for continued certification termed the Professional Development Portfolio (PDP).[42–45] To maintain registered status, RDN/RDs and NDTR/DTRs must participate in the CDR's mandatory PDP recertification system and remit the annual registration maintenance fee. Using this plan, the individual RDN/RD and NDTR/DTR assumes the responsibility for learning, professional development, and career direction. The PDP requires each practitioner to first engage in self-reflection, followed by assessment and goal setting. This process is followed by the development of a 5-year plan that reflects a critical analysis of goals and the steps to be taken to maintain professional competency. The Academy's "Revised 2012 Standards of Practice in Nutrition Care and Standards of Professional Performance for Registered Dietitians" and the CDR's "Professional Development Portfolio" mutually ensure competence of the dietetics practitioner.[46,47] See https//www.cdrnet.org.

As greater numbers of registered dietitians retire, maintaining competence and adhering to the Code of Ethics for the Profession of Dietetics will present challenges, especially for those maintaining RDN/RD status.[48] A recent article by Dahl and Nye discusses this issue, which could be viewed as relevant to all practitioners in detail.[49]

Participation in continuing professional education activities is essential for lifelong development to maintain and improve knowledge and skills for competent dietetics practice. RDN/RDs and NDRT/DTRs must report continuing professional education activities CPEU) using the portfolio recertification system. The process by which the required 75 CPEUs are accumulated is also determined by the CDR, which specifies the educational activities that qualify to be used as CPEUs. Beginning with the 5-year recertification starting in 2012 and ending in 2017, RDs and DTRs are required to complete 1 CPEU in ethics (Learning Need Code 1050). The details of the continuing education requirements including the new ethics requirement can be accessed at https://www .cdrnet.org.

To maintain certification, an RDN/RD is required to pay yearly maintenance fee and engage in 75 hours of continuing education (CPEU) over a 5-year period. A DTR/NDTR pays yearly fee and must accrue 50 hours (CPEU) in a 5-year period. The details for dietitians and technicians maintaining certification can be found at the CDR website (https://www .cdrnet.org) under the Professional Development Resource Center.

RECERTIFICATION OF SPECIALISTS AND ADVANCED PRACTICE IN CLINICAL NUTRITION

The specialty board certification is a practice credential (just as RDN/RD and DTR/NDTR) that represents to the public that the certificate holder possesses the knowledge, skills, and experience to function effectively as a specialist in a specific focus area of practice. The nature of the knowledge and skills to practice at a specialty level is subject to change due to technological and scientific advances. Recertification testing helps to provide continuing assurance that the certified specialist has indeed maintained knowledge in his or her specialty or focus area. Details of the recertification process for each specialist can be found at the following link: https://www.cdrnet.org.

Therefore, those who wish to recertify in the same specialty area at the end of their 5-year certification period must meet the following criteria:

- Currently be a registered dietitian with the CDR
- Successfully complete an eligibility application
- Submit an application fee
- Successfully complete a specialty examination

APPROPRIATE USE OF CREDENTIALS

In 1989, the CDR issued a statement on the protection of the credentials RD and DTR.[50] The CDR recognized that the credentials that it controls are most valuable to it and to the holders of those credentials because they are awarded only to individuals who have met the education and experiential requirements and have passed appropriate examinations. Practitioners may use these credentials only if they continue to meet CDR requirements, including payment of a registration maintenance fee and fulfillment of the continuing education hours required. The 2009 Code of Ethics for the Profession of Dietetics has specific details about the use of the various credentials of the Academy of Nutrition and Dietetics along with responsibilities and consequences.[51]

As noted in the CDR statement, "The most common usage is after the practitioner's name as a professional designation, e.g., Jane Doe, RD or John Smith, DTR."[52] Other specific details of the joint policy statement of the CDR and the Academy's board of directors are available online at: https://www.cdrnet.org.

LEGAL REGULATION STATUTES FOR DIETITIANS NUTRITIONISTS AND DIETETIC TECHNICIANS

Forty-seven states and Puerto Rico now have laws that regulate dietitians or nutritionists through licensure, statutory certification, or registration. Thirty-eight, or 80 percent, of these states have included the protection of a scope of practice as well as protection of the name registered dietitian. One-half of these states protect the title of nutritionist as well; Nebraska protects the title of medical nutrition therapist, and Maine has licensure for dietetic technicians. State licensure and state certification are entirely separate and distinct from registration or certification by the CDR (https://www.cdrnet.org).

The 47 states that regulate dietitians or nutritionists do so through licensure, statutory certification, or registration. For state regulation purposes, these terms are defined as the following:[53]

- *Licensure.* Licensure is a process by which state governmental agencies grant time-limited permission to an individual to be recognized as and/or engaged in a given occupation after verifying that the individual has met predetermined, standardized competency qualifications.
- *Statutory certification.* This certification limits use of particular titles to persons meeting predetermined requirements, while persons not certified can still practice the occupation or profession.

- *Registration.* It is the least restrictive form of state regulation. As with certification, unregistered persons are permitted to practice the profession. Typically, exams are not given and enforcement of the registration requirement is minimal.

Dietetic practitioners are licensed by states to ensure that only qualified, trained professionals provide nutrition services or advice to individuals requiring or seeking nutrition care or dietetics information. In states with licensure, only state-licensed dietetics professionals can provide nutrition counseling and other services, included in the scope of practice, as a part of the licensure law. Non-licensed practitioners may be subject to prosecution for practicing without a license. States with certification laws limit the use of particular titles (e.g., dietitian or nutritionist) to persons meeting predetermined requirements; however, persons not certified can still practice without using the title. Consumers in these states who are seeking nutrition therapy assistance need to be more cautious and aware of the qualifications of the provider they choose.

As dietitian nutritionists or dietetic technicians travel from state to state to practice dietetics, it is important to contact a state Academy of Nutrition and Dietetics or a state regulatory agency to determine state licensure law provisions prior to practicing dietetics. Contacting the state Academy or State licensure agency will provide specific state related information about licensure in the state. CDR maintains a current list of states with licensure and or certification laws as well (https://www.cdrnet.org).

SUMMARY

Dietitians continue to desire recognition and differentiation among their peers that is visible and can be communicated to consumers, clients, and other professional practitioners. The CDR credentialing program does this. The RDN/RD has become valued to the point that most individuals consider it synonymous with dietitian. The same is becoming true for the DTR/NDTR. Many employers view both as mandatory credentials to practice in various employment settings for dietetic professionals. Credentials also have been used in international markets and jobs to describe individuals and job qualifications. For dietitians, dietetic technicians, and dietetic specialists, this is a plus as the world moves toward a global practice and global economy.

Consumers will always demand credentials of some kind. As consumers recognize that the credentials of the Commission on Dietetic Registration provide assurance that the practitioners are competent and can provide services they want, the demand will continue to rise. More significantly, these credentials will enhance the dietetics professionals' efforts to describe the diversity of their capabilities and to obtain a competitive advantage in the practice of dietetics in the United States and internationally.

DEFINITIONS

Certification. The process by which a nongovernmental agency or association grants recognition to an individual who has met certain predetermined qualifications specified by that agency or association (e.g., registration for dietitians and dietetic technicians administered by the CDR).

Credentialing. Formal recognition of professional or technical competence as by certification or licensure.

Licensure. Process by which a government agency grants permission to an individual to engage in a given occupation upon finding that the applicant has attained the minimal degree of competency necessary to ensure that the public health, safety, and welfare are reasonably well protected.

Practitioner. One who practices in a profession or occupation.

Registration. See Certification.

Scope of practice. Extent of or dimensions of activities performed in an area of practice.

For additional definitions of terms commonly used by the Academy consult the 2016 Updated Definition of Terms List.[54]

REFERENCES

1. Commission on Dietetic Registration: Accessed April 11, 2016, https://www.cdrnet.org
2. Cassell, J. *Carry the Flame: The History of the American Dietetic Association.* (Chicago: The American Dietetic Association, 1990), p. 9.
3. See Note 2, p. 3.
4. Academy of Dietetics and Nutrition Quality Management Committee. Definition of Terms List. Updated January 2015. Accessed April 11, 2016, https:/www.eatrightpro.org/_/media/eatrightpro%20files/practice/scope%20standards%20of%20practice/definition%20of%20of20terms%20list.ashx

5. See Note 2, p. 22.
6. See Note 2, p. 26.
7. See Note 2, p. 71.
8. Perry, E. "Report of the Executive Board." *J Am Diet Assoc* 26 (1950): 949–957.
9. ADA. *Constitution of the American Dietetic Association, as Amended.* (Chicago: The American Dietetic Association, 1971).
10. Bogle, M.L. "Registration: The *Sine Qua Non* of a Competent Dietitian." *J Am Diet Assoc* 74 (1974): 616–620.
11. See Note 1.
12. ADA. "Bylaws of American Dietetic Association," revised March 10, 2002. Accessed March 1, 2004, www.eatright.org/member/governance/85_12428.cfm
13. ADA. "American Dietetic Association/Commission on Dietetic Registration Code of Ethics for the Profession of Dietetics and Process for Consideration of Ethics Issues." *J Am Diet Assoc* 109 (2009): 1461–1467.
14. ADA. *Council on Future Practice Visioning Report.* (Chicago: The American *Dietetic Association*, 2011).
15. See Note 13.
16. The Academy Quality Management Committee and Scope of Practice Subcommittee of The Quality Management Committee. "Academy of Nutrition and Dietetics: Scope of Practice for the Registered Dietitian." *J Acad Nutr Diet* 113, no. 6 (2013): S17–S28.
17. The Academy Quality Management Committee and Scope of Practice Subcommittee of the Quality Management Committee. "Academy of Nutrition and Dietetics: Revised 2012 Standards of Practice in Nutrition Care and Standards of Professional Performance for Registered Dietitians." *J Acad Nutr Diet* 113, no. 6 (2013): S29–S45.
18. The Academy Quality Management Committee and Scope of Practice Subcommittee of the Quality Management Committee. "Academy of Nutrition and Dietetics: Scope of Practice for the Dietitian Technician, Registered." *J Acad Nutr Diet* 113, no. 6 (2013): S46–S55.
19. See Note 18.
20. The Academy Quality Management Committee and Scope of Practice Subcommittee of the Quality Management Committee. "Academy of Nutrition and Dietetics: Revised 2012 Standards of Practice in Nutrition Care and Standards of Professional Performance for the Dietetic Technician, Registered." *J Acad Nutr Diet* 113, no. 6 (2013): S56–S71.
21. ADA. *Final Report of the Phase 2 Future Practice and Education Task Force.* (Chicago: The American Dietetic Association, 2008), pp. 2–72.
22. See Note 21.
23. Dreyfus, H.L., and S.E. Dreyfus. *Mind over Machine.* (New York: The Free Press, 1986).
24. Dreyfus, S.E. "The Five-Stage Model of Adult Skill Acquisition." *Bull Sci Technol Soc* 14 (2004): 177–181.
25. See Note 13.

26. See Note 18.
27. See Note 20.
28. See Note 4.
29. Raynor, H.A., and C.M. Champagne. "Position of the Academy of Nutrition and Dietetics Interventions for the Treatment of Overweight and Obesity in Adults." *J Acad Nutr Diet* 116, no. 1 (2016): 129–147.
30. Bogle, M.L., L. Balogun, J. Cassell, A. Catakis, H.J. Holler, and C. Flynn. "Achieving Excellence in Dietetic Practice: Certification of Specialists and Advanced-level Practitioners." *J Am Diet Assoc* 93 (1993): 149–150.
31. Touger-Decker, R. "Advanced-level Practice Degree Options: Practice Doctorates in Dietetics." *J Am Diet Assoc* 104 (2004): 1456–1458.
32. Skipper, A., and N.M. Lewis. "Using Initiative to Achieve Autonomy: A Model for Advanced Practice in Medical Mutrition Therapy." *J Am Diet Assoc* 106 (2006): 1219–1225.
33. Academy of Nutrition and Dietetics. *Visioning Report: Moving Forward—A Vision for the Continuum of Dietetics Education, Credentialing and Practice.* (Chicago, IL: Academy of Nutrition and Dietetics, 2012). Accessed April 11, 2016, http://www .eatrightpro.org/~/media/eatrightpro%20files/practice/future%20practice /visioning%20report%20final.ashx
34. Commission on Dietetic Registration. "Commission on Dietetic Registration 2005–2007 Levels of Practice Study Executive Summary." Accessed April 11, 2016, https://www.cdrnet.org/whatsnew/Executive%20Summary.htm
35. Brody, R.A., L. Byham-Gray, M.R. Passannante, R. Touger-Decker, and J. O'Sullivan-Maillet. "Essential Practice Activities of Clinical Advanced Practice Registered Dietitians: A Delphi Study." *J Am Diet Assoc* 111 (2011): A17.
36. Brody, R.A., L. Byham-Gray, R. Touger-Decker, M.R. Passannante, and J. O'Sullivan Malliet. "Identifying Components of Advanced-clinical Nutrition Practice: A Delphi Study." *J Am Diet Assoc* 112 (1012): 859–869.
37. Wildish, D.E., S. Evers. "A Definition, Description, and Framework for Advanced Practice in Dietetics." *Can J Diet Pract Res* 71, no. 1 (2010): ed–e11.
38. O'Sullivan Maillet, J., R.A. Brody, A Skipper, J.M. Pavlinac. "Framework for Analyzing Supply and Demand for Specialist and Advanced Practice Registered Dietitians." *J Acad Nutr Diet* 112, 3 suppl (2012): S47–S55.
39. Brody, R.A., L. Byham-Gray, R. Touger-Decker, M.R. Passannante, P. Rothpletz-Puglia, J. O'Sullivan Maillet. "What Clinical Activities Do Advanced Practice Registered Dietitians Nutritionists Perform? Results of a Delphi Study." *J Acad Nutr Diet* 114, no. 5 (2014): 718–733.
40. Mueller, C., D. Rogers, R.A. Brody, C.L. Chaffee Jr, R. Tougher-Decker. "Report from the Advanced-Level Clinical Practice Audit Task Force of the Commission on Dietetic Registration: Results of the 2013 Advanced-Level Clinical Practice Audit." *J Acad Nutr Diet* 115, no. 4 (2015): 624–634.
41. Brody, R.A., A. Skipper, C.L. Chaffee Jr, N.H. Wooldridge, J.R. Kicklighter, R. Tougher-Decker. "Developing an Advanced Practice Credential for Registered Dietitian Nutritionists in Clinical Nutrition Practice." *J Acad Nutr Diet* 115, no. 4 (2015): 619–623.

42. Weddle, D.O., S.P. Himsburg, N. Collins, and R. Lewis. "The Professional Development Portfolio Process: Setting Goals for Credentialing." *J Am Diet Assoc* 102, no. 10 (2002): 1439–1444.

43. See Note 4, p. 4.

44. Keirn, K.S., C.A. Johnson, and G.E. Gates. "Learning Needs and Continuing Professional Education Activities of Professional Development Portfolio Participants." *J Am Diet Assoc* 101, no. 6 (2001): 697–702.

45. Keirn, K.S., G.E. Gates, and C.A. Johnson. "Dietetics Professionals Have a Positive Perception of Professional Development." *J Am Diet Assoc* 101, no. 7 (2001): 820–824.

46. See Note 17.

47. See Note 42.

48. Gates, G. "Ethics Opinion: Dietetic Professionals Are Ethically Obligated to Maintain Personal Competence in Practice." *J Am Diet Assoc* 103 (2003): 633–635.

49. Dahl, L., and S. Nye. "Competency for Retired Credentialed Practitioners." *J Am Diet Assoc* 112 (2012): 934–936.

50. Academy of Nutrition and Dietetics. "RD/DTR Credentialing (CDR)." Accessed April 11, 2016, http://www.eatright.org/HealthProfessionals/content.aspx?id=64 42458781&terms=RD%2fDTR%20Credentialing#.UPsWAI5xBFA

51. See Note 13.

52. See Note 50.

53. See Note 4.

54. Ibid.

CHAPTER 5

The Nutrition and Dietetics Professional

"The dietetics practitioner provides professional services with objectivity and with respect for the unique needs and values of individuals."[1]

OUTLINE

LEARNING OBJECTIVES

The student will be able to:
1. Become familiar with Scope of Practice and its implications for the Academy member.
2. Understand the attributes of a professional.
3. Become familiar with the essential elements of ethical practice and the Code of Ethics.
4. Gain appreciation for the importance of lifelong professional development.
5. Know how to apply evidence-based practice.

INTRODUCTION

Professional practice can be defined in several ways—first and foremost as practice based on specialized learning and training and adherence to a code of ethical actions and behavior adopted by the group. Dietitians who develop a professional portfolio are familiar with the process involved, such as a plan for continued competence in practice with supporting goals and measures to meet the goals. The portfolio emphasis is on continued learning and self-monitoring—both distinguishing features of a professional.

Dietetics practice is based on a fluid and flexible framework. The core of the profession is food and nutrition services for individuals, groups, and communities. The dietetics professional provides services through communication and collaboration with others by using management techniques, research, science, technology, and leadership skills.

SCOPE OF PRACTICE AND PERFORMANCE STANDARDS

In response to a need to provide guidance for members practicing in diverse roles in dietetics, the Academy appointed a Task Force in 2004 to develop a Scope of Practice Framework. Directions for using the framework followed with periodic updates. The framework provided a flexible decision-making structure by which dietitians could determine if specific activities fell within the scope of dietetics practice. Three broad areas were defined in the framework: foundation knowledge, evaluation, and resources.

Scope of Practice (Individual) is also referred to as Scope of Practice in Nutrition and Dietetics and provides the flexible boundaries of the individual's professional practice. For the Scope of Practice (Statutory) the Academy has adopted the definition of the Center for the Health Professions, University of California, San Francisco. It can be accessed at http://future .ucsf.edu/Content/29/2007-12 Promising Scope of Practice Models for the Health professions.pdf. The statutory Scope of Practice refers to the practitioner's qualifications, board representation, fees, and renewal as well as listing a range of roles, examples of specific activities and regulations within which the nutrition and dietetics practitioners perform.[2] The scope of practice for the registered dietitian nutritionist (RDN) focuses on "food and nutrition and related service developed, directed and provided by RDNs to protect the public, community, and populations; enhance the health and well-being of patients/clients; and deliver quality products, programs, and services across all focus areas."[3] The scope of practice for the dietetic technician, registered (DTR) focuses on "food and nutrition-related services provided by DTRs who work under supervision when in direct patient/client nutrition care and who may work independently."[4] As a part of the Scope of Practice, the Standards of Practice (SOP) and the Standards of Professional Performance (SOPP) are used as tools by credentialed dietetics practitioners. They are to be used for self-evaluation, professional development, and advancement of practice. Some regulatory agencies may use the SOP and SOPP to determine competency for credentialed practitioners.[5]

Standards of Practice and Standards of Professional Performance

The Academy published guidelines for professional practice in 1998 and revised them in 2012 as "Scope of Practice in Nutrition and Dietetics."[6] The first standards for a specific or focus area were developed for the Registered Dietitian and Dietetic Technician in nutrition care and revised in 2012.[7,8] They were general in content that outlined activities that apply in all areas of dietetic practice. These became the blueprint for the development of standards in many other areas of practice. The general standards specified the following activities:

- Minimum levels of practice and performance
- Common indicators for self-evaluation
- Consistency in practice and performance
- The role of dietetics and the services that the RDN and the DTR provide within the healthcare team

- The food and nutrition services provided in a framework that encourages continuous quality improvement
- A basis for researchers to investigate relationships between dietetics practice and outcomes
- A framework for educators to set objectives for educational programs that reflect applicable federal laws and regulations

Professional standards are important because they promote safe, effective, and efficient food and nutrition services; they are developed from evidence-based practice (EBP); they provide for improved health care and food and nutrition service-related outcomes; they ensure continuous quality improvement; they promote dietetics research, innovation, and practice development, and they help the individual RDN and DTR develop professionally.

SOP and SOPP have now been developed in many areas of dietetic practice. SOP can be defined as "the minimum expectations or skill for competent performance". SOPP may be defined as "guides for the activities regarded as essential to attain professional expectations that is, the knowledge, skills, and competencies required at various levels of care." In simplest terms, the SOP describes what is done—the job requirements—at defined levels of skill and the SOPP describes the actions necessary to achieve this. The two are complementary documents and are developed to be used together.

The following areas of practice have developed SOP and SOPP documents, which are available on the Academy website and in the Journal of the Academy.

a. Adult Weight Management
b. Pediatrics
c. Public Health and Community Nutrition
d. Sustainable, Resilient, and healthy Food and Water Systems
e. Sports Nutrition
f. Management in Food and Nutrition Systems
g. Nephrology Nutrition
h. Nutrition Support
i. Nutrition Care for Registered Dietitians
j. Nutrition Care for Dietetic Technicians
k. Clinical Nutrition Management
l. Intellectual and Developmental Disabilities
m. Disordered Eating and Eating Disorders

n. Diabetes Care
o. Integrative and Functional Medicine
p. Extended Care Settings
q. Oncology Nutrition Care
r. Education of Dietetics Practitioners
s. Diabetes
t. Behavioral Health Care

In addition to the standards for areas of practice, standards have also been developed by the Academy for organization self-assessment and quality improvement.[9]

ETHICAL PRACTICE

The *Code of Ethics for the Profession of Dietetics* is the guiding document for ethical practice. The Code is developed by the Academy and the Council for Dietetic Registration as a voluntary enforceable code of behavior. The code challenges all members to uphold ethical principles. The process of enforcement includes a way to deal with any complaints about members and credentialed practitioners. An ethics committee enforces the code and educated members about the ethical principles to be followed.

Several guiding principles outline the concerns, values and ethics of the dietetics profession as follows:[10]

1. The nutrition and dietetics practitioner conducts himself or herself with honesty, integrity, and fairness.
2. The nutrition and dietetics practitioner supports and promotes high standards of professional practice. The practitioner accepts the obligation to protect clients, the public, and the profession by upholding the Code of Ethics and reporting perceived violations of the Code through the processes provided.
3. The practitioner provides professional services with objectivity and with respect and consideration for the unique needs and values of individuals.
4. The practitioner protects confidential information and makes full disclosure about any limitations to guarantee full confidentiality.
5. The practitioner does not invite, accept or offer gifts, monetary incentives, or other considerations that affect or reasonably give an appearance of affecting his or her professional judgment.

6. The nutrition and dietetics practitioner does not invite, accept or offer gifts, monetary incentives, or other considerations that affect or reasonably give an appearance of affecting his or her professional judgment.

In all areas of practice, situations arise at times in which the ethical course of action may not always be clear. Ethical conflicts of interest and poorly conducted business practices are examples of how unethical conduct may impact dietetic practice.[11] Other ethical considerations include issues of confidentiality, promotion and endorsement of products, and recognition of professional judgment.

In clinical practice, activities relating to providing dietary supplementation advice and conducting online counseling and consultation make it important to be familiar with regulations as well as the code of ethics in order to avoid liability risk. Other instances in which ethical conduct must be considered are disclosure of confidential information, accepting gifts, discussing patient/clients, and charting or giving information about prices or salaries. In such cases, open discussion with a supervisor or trusted experienced peers, checking relevant policies before acting is the best course to follow. A personal code of conduct that espouses integrity, fairness, and a sense of always wanting to do the right thing helps make difficult decisions about ethical questions easier.

The increased use of electronic communications in all areas of practice requires ethical decision-making.[12] There are few guidelines for the use of media that deal with ethical behavior and communication with the public and it is often difficult to know what is reliable and valid information. The Nutrition Entrepreneurship Dietetic Practice group has established a nutrition blog to make it easier to find science-based information and elevate the voice of the registered dietitian online.[13] *E-professionalism* is a term used to describe professional attitudes and behaviors in the use of digital media and applies to still-evolving SOP, legality etiquette, and perception.[14]

Ethics in research and the use of copyrighted material from journals are also areas in which dietitians need to be aware of regulations that apply and use professional judgment.[15]

The obligation to maintain personal competence in practice is emphasized as an ethical obligation.[16] Practitioners need to continually build on their knowledge and skills and to continue to acquire new techniques and evidence-based information. By continuing to stay current, improved performance provides quality service in the work setting.

The manager or leader assists in developing organization practices and policies that promote ethical practice. Such policies set the ethical standards for activities, such as purchasing, financial management, patient care, and information provided to patients and clients. The manager or leader sets an example for ethical behavior built on openness and trust and makes sure all employees know the policies and procedures of the workplace. The manager assists in making ethical decisions by identifying that the situation is an ethical dilemma, determining how the issue applies to the Code of Ethics, and selecting alternative actions and strategies to successfully implement a decision.[17]

An ethical deliberation process is shown in **Table 5-1.**

Table 5-1.   Suggested Ethical Deliberative Process

1. Clarify the moral question—the first statement of the moral problem
2. Re-create the context.
   a. Gather data.
   b. Consider relevant facts.
   c. Consider relevant values.
3. Name stakeholders and their relationships.
4. Identify ways of ethical thinking used by the stakeholder.
   a. Rules thinking—doing what is right by following the rules
   b. Role thinking—being true to self and your sense of virtue
   c. Goals thinking—producing good outcomes regardless of rules
5. Determine practical limits to the situation: policies, laws, standards, and codes.
6. Balance a client's belief and preferences with his or her best interests.
7. Respect advance directives.
8. Assume a client has decisional capacity.
9. If not, select a substitute decision maker if necessary.
10. Restate the ethical problem.
11. Search for possible options
12. Test various options. Check through each option for:
    a. Rules—is it right?
    b. Roles—can I feel good about this?
    c. Goal—what good will it do?
13. Justify the option selected for recommendation.
    a. Keep the client's best interest at the center of options.
    b. Provide a description of what will likely happen and provide a clear action.
    c. Plan for each option recommended—suggestions of practical pathways.

Reprinted from Journal of the American Dietetic Association, 102, Number 5 (May 2002): Julie O'Sullivan Maillet et al, "Position of the American Dietetic Association: Ethical and Legal Issues in Nutrition, Hydration, and Feeding," 716–726, Copyright 2002, with permission from Elsevier.

DIVERSITY AND CULTURALLY COMPETENT PRACTICE

A former president of the Academy described culturally competent practice as a way to overcome health disparities and improve care across all population groups.[18] Interaction with clients of diverse cultures in a sensitive and effective manner is a key strategy in the promotion of food and nutrition behavior and beliefs.

Cultural competence is often implemented through diversity initiatives. Diversity can refer to age, physical ability, religion, socioeconomic status, sex, and ethnicity. Professional organizations sensitive to diversity issues focus on attracting a membership that reflects these demographics.[19] The Academy has developed a number of initiatives toward promoting diversity, including the following official statement: "The Academy values and respects the diverse viewpoints and individual differences of all people. The Academy's mission and vision are most effectively realized through the promotion of a diverse membership that reflects cultural, ethnic, gender, race, religious, sexual orientation, socioeconomic, geographical, political, educational, experiential and philosophical characteristics of the public it serves. The Academy actively identifies and offers opportunities to individuals with varied skills, talents, abilities, ideas, disabilities, backgrounds, and practice expertise."[20]

The Code of Ethics further delineates issues relating to ensuring equality in practice. Reflecting the Academy's commitment to diversity, several grants and awards are provided by the profession. These include Diversity Mini-Grants for students and underrepresented groups within the profession and Diversity Promotion Grants to support minority recruitment and retention projects. The Diversity Leaders Program supports active members from underrepresented groups within the profession and a Diversity Action Award to an educational institution, Affiliate dietetic association, dietetic practice group, or other recognized Academy group in recognition of past accomplishments. A compilation of articles published in a Journal Supplement is titled: "Building a Brighter Tomorrow: Diversity, Mentoring, and the Future of Dietetics."[21]

LIFELONG PROFESSIONAL DEVELOPMENT

The Center for Professional Development in the Academy office offers and coordinates activities designed to support all food and nutrition professionals in continual building of their knowledge and skills. The activities include multidisciplinary topics, enhanced technology skills, and programming. Examples are the annual Food and Nutrition Conference and Exposition (FNCE); training programs for specialty certification and conferences and events including sessions at FNCE conducted by dietetic practice groups. Build distance-learning opportunities are also offered through teleseminars and webinars. In addition, group and individual self-study is available.

Delivery of Learning

Food and nutrition professionals use a variety of methods to continually build professional skills. The range of learning opportunities is greater than ever considering the many advancements in technology that allow individual study a well as group learning and interaction. For example, teleconferencing today replaces many former face-to-face meetings, thus saving travel and related costs. Networking through social network sites is another way dietetic professionals connect with and learn from others with similar interests and concerns.[22]

Online video and streaming video are effective ways of communicating nutrition messages.[23] Switt[24] offers suggestions for creating and managing a website by offering unique, original content; registering with search engines, and developing a newsletter.

Self-direction in learning is the ability to engage in educational activities without external reinforcement. Individuals who do so typify some or all of the following characteristics:

- Willingness to change
- Ability to identify weaknesses or shortcomings
- Ability to capitalize on strengths
- Ability to learn from constructive criticism
- Willingness to participate in all forms of learning
- Willingness to try new techniques for learning
- Willingness to invest time and money in learning
- Willingness to find a mentor or become one
- Volunteering in organizations and groups
- Sharing learning by applying concepts with others
- Providing feedback to instructors, mentors and supervisors
- Assuming personal responsibility for learning
- Allowing the possibility of new careers and experiences

Besides maintaining and improving professional competence, there are other reasons for participation in continuing education activities and why there may be deterrents in doing so. Several reasons and deterrents are shown in **Table 5-2.** To determine the types of learning experiences that most benefit an individual, several questions may be posed for self-examination of needs (**Table 5-3**).

Informatics

Informatics refers to the use of electronic support for using and managing information. Health informatics is described by the Department of Health and Human Services as "the intersection of information science, computer media, and health care." Health information tools include electronic media, clinical guidelines, formal medical technologies, and information and communication systems. The medical and nursing professions have taken the lead in the use of technology, most directly in the development of electronic health records.[25]

Nutrition informatics is defined as "the effective retrieval, organization, storage, and optimum use of information, data, and knowledge of food

---

Table 5-2. Factors Influencing Continuing Professional Education

Reasons for participation in continuing professional education:
- Professional development and improvement
- Professional service
- College learning and interaction
- Professional commitment and reflection
- Personal benefits and job security

Deterrents to participation in continuing professional education:
- Disengagement and apathy for learning or career
- Costs
- Family
- Failure to see the worth or benefit
- Lack of quality in offerings
- Demands of work constraints

Reprinted from Journal of the American Dietetic Association, 103, Number 3 (March 2003), Petrillo, T. "Lifelong Learning Goals: Individual Steps That Propel the Profession of Dietetics," 298–300, Copyright 2003, with permission from Elsevier.

Table 5-3.   Questions to Determine Self-Needs

What kind of learning is needed to improve performance in your current job?

How can you change or improve your current job?

What is your capacity for learning and growth in a new job?

What transferable skills do you possess for a new career path?

What new skills are required for you to be qualified to contribute in a new job?

What are your personal interests?

What career path did you once consider?

What leisure time interests do you enjoy?

What type of a learning experience is most favorable to you and why?

What related learning opportunities lie just beyond your field of practice?

What skill sets are important to your employer?

Data from Davis, J.R. *Toolbox for Reflection and Developing an Action Learning Plan: Managing Your Own.* (San Francisco: Berrett-Koehler Publisher 2000), p. 10. Petrillo, T. "Lifelong Learning Goals: Individual Steps That Propel the Profession of Dietetics." *J Am Diet Assoc* 103, no. 3 (2003): 298–300.

and nutrition-related problem solving and decision making." Informatics is supported by the use of information standards, information processing and information technology.[26] The term is also simply defined as "the intersection of information, nutrition, and technology." The use of automation is transforming dietetic practice in hospital dietary departments as well as in business, research, and private practice. The time involved in nutrition assessments of patients can be decreased, communications between clinical and food service areas can be accomplished much faster. Dietitians can help shape the trend toward automation in hospitals and food service institutions. The demand for informatics is expected to continue to grow, making this an area in which dietitians need to become proficient.[27]

Dietitians use websites for information that is scientifically sound and that provides information from many sources. Foremost among these is the Academy Evidence Analysis Library.[28]

A national undertaking that will connect health records to electronics for every American is under way. The dietetics profession is a part of the national effort, making it imperative that a concerted effort is made to prepare practitioners for the use of nutrition information aligned with the broad fields of medicine and health. This also presents the opportunity to integrate food and nutrition with related activities into the system.[29]

Health Insurance Portability and Accountability Act

All practitioners need to be familiar with the provisions of the Health Insurance Portability and Accountability Act (HIPPA) Act of 1996 and the additional Privacy Rule of 2003.[30] Developed by the Department of Health and Human Services, these acts provide patients with access to their medical records and increased control over their health information. HIPPA includes provisions for electronic transactions and safeguards to protect the security and confidentiality of health information. All health providers, including dietitians, must be aware of the need to protect the privacy of information about patients in the clinical setting and be familiar with the policies and procedures established by the institution for the enforcement of the regulations.[31]

THE LEGAL BASIS OF PRACTICE

The practice of dietetics is directly affected by many laws and regulations that must be followed in order to avoid legal consequences. Fortunately, as Derelian[32] points out, almost all disputes that involve a dietitian would be of a civil nature, such as contract breaches or negligence. Busey[33] indicates that dietitians may increasingly become parties to lawsuits considering the number of RDNs who go into private practice and the fact that they play important roles in the healthcare process. He gives suggestions regarding the types of lawsuits in which a dietitian may become involved and discusses steps in the process when lawsuits occur. He further points out that if the terminology used in documentation of patient care is subject to more than one interpretation, this could become a legally disputed issue. An example is the use of the word *inadequate* in describing patient progress, as it could denote negligence.[34]

Three specific areas of practice that are of importance regarding possible legal issues are: practice beyond one's qualifications, billing, and proper use of healthcare resources and advertising services.[35] Responsibility in practice can mean that as advanced tasks become part of the job requirements, additional training will usually be needed. Examples are in activities such as insulin regulation, diet ordering, and placement of a nasal gastric tube. Similarly, if the dietitian advances in job level, further credentials, and learning may be required.

Dietitians working in clinical practice as well as in business or private practice need to develop and use standardized billing procedures, including written documents that explain the billing to clients. Billing to third party payers will always entail policies and procedures that must be adhered to in order to avoid legal complications.

Registered dietitians who advertise their services must be honest in all claims made and should list their areas of preferred or limited practice. Claims for guaranteed results should never be made if he or she is unable to document the results. All practices should be sound—nutritionally, ethically, and legally.

The increased use of electronic technology such as in telehealth or telemedicine in which the dietitian may be a participant is another area in which legal questions may arise.[36] Examples of such issues are licensure, facility certification and accreditation, reimbursement and Medicare Part B issues, and professional liability insurance. All dietitians are strongly encouraged to carry personal liability insurance for protection against malpractice or other issues described.

EVIDENCE-BASED PRACTICE

EBP is viewed as necessary for the best outcomes in all areas of dietetic practice. Evidence-based medicine is a model of clinical decision-making that uses a systematic process to integrate the best research-based evidence with clinical expertise and patient values to answer questions about a patient's plan of care.[36] EBP is described as "the use of systematically reviewed scientific evidence in making food and nutrition practice decisions by integrating the best available evidence with professional expertise and client values to improve outcomes."[37] Dietitians need to incorporate EBP into activities as payment for services may be dependent on outcomes. Change in practice is constant, and this approach ensures that decisions are sound. By applying the process, dietitians are able to successfully compete in the healthcare environment where positive outcomes, proven efficiency, cost effectiveness, and sharing of outcomes are important.

The Academy provides a valuable resource to members through the Evidence Analysis Library (EAL). Through use of the EAL, professionals can stay current on the research in any area of dietetics. A variety of resources are offered, including evidence summaries of the major research on any given topic, bibliographies, and conclusion statements with an evaluation of the strength of the evidence.[37]

A guide for appraising resources for evidence-based information is shown in **Table 5-4**. Evidence must be balanced with the client's values and preferences for optimal shared decision-making, and resources must be reliable, relevant, and readable.[38]

Table 5-4. Guide for Appraising Resources for Evidence-Based Information

Method and quality of information

- How was the resource compiled?
- Were explicit criteria for seeking and appraising evidence described, and were they adhered to?
- How is the resource maintained?

Rating scale for methods and quality of information

0. No evidence cited

1. Evidence is cited, but there is no explicit criteria for the selection or evaluation of the content; the selection of content suggests lack of consistent evidence standards

2. Evidence is cited, and there are explicit criteria for the election or evaluation of the content, or both the selection of content suggests lack of adherence to these evidence standards.

3. Evident is cited, but there are not explicit criteria for the selection or evaluation of the content the selection of content suggests adherence to some evidence standards.

4. Evidence is cited, and there are explicit criteria for the selection or evaluation of the content, or both; the selection of content suggests some adherence to evidence standards.

5. Evidence I cited, and there are explicit criteria for the selection and evaluation of the content the selection of content suggest adherence to evidence standards most of the time.

Clinical usefulness

- Did the resource provide clinically useful answers?
- How did you use this resource?
- Was it easy to use?
- Were the answers easily accessible and readable within a few minutes?
- Will you use this resource?
- If so, when and how?

Rating scale for clinical usefulness

0. Not useful clinically.

1. Clinically useful answers are rarely available and are not easily accessible or readable within a few minutes.

2. Clinically useful answers are available some of the time but are not easily accessible or readable within a few minutes.

3. Clinically useful answers are available some of the time and are easily accessible and readable within a few minutes.

4. Clinically useful answers are available most of the time but are not easily accessible or readable within a few minutes.

5. Clinically useful answers are available most of the time and are easily accessible and readable within a few minutes.

Table 5-4. Guide for Appraising Resources for Evidence-Based Information (Continued)

Details on specific resources

Evidence-based medical texts

The following points could be used as a minimal checklist:

- Does the resource provide an explicit statement about the type of evidence on which any statements or recommendation are based? Did the authors adhere to these criteria? For example, claims about effectiveness of an intervention might be accompanied by a statement about either the level of evidence (which would need to be defined somewhere in the text) or a statement about the exact type of evidence (e.g., "There have been three randomized controlled trials.")

- Was there an explicit and adequate search for this evidence? For example, a search for evidence about an intervention might have started with a look for adequate systematic reviews. If this was done, it might be followed by a search of the Cochrane Central Register of Controlled Trials.

- Is there quantification of the results? For example, statements about diagnostic accuracy should contain measures of accuracy such as sensitivity and specificity.

The minimum criteria for an evidence-based resource would be adherence to the first bullet point. Better resources should also address the other two points.

Meta-resources (e.g., listings or search engines for other resources)

These resources should provide and explicit statement about the selection criteria for inclusion in the listing. Better resource should also include a descriptive review such as that described in the three points for evidence-based medical texts.

SUMMARY

The professional dietitian is one who is competent in practice and continually participates in ongoing education. Knowledge and skills go hand in hand with personal qualities and ethical practice, understanding the legal basis of practice and incorporating the concept of evidence-based activities in professional practice. As the voice of authority in food and nutrition, the dietitian is a professional in every sense of the term.

DEFINITIONS

Diversity. A term with multiple, subjective definitions; may refer to age, physical ability, religion, socioeconomic status, sex, race, ethnicity, or other factors.

Evidence-based. Action based on research data and evaluation of outcomes.

Standard. A measure of proficiency at an established level.

REFERENCES

1. Code of Ethics for the Profession of Dietetics and Process for Consideration of Ethics Issues.
2. Definition of Terms List. Academy of Nutrition and Dietetics. Approved by House of Delegates Leadership Team January 27, 2016.
3. Scope of Practice in Nutrition and Dietetics. "Academy Quality Management Committee and Scope of Practice Subcommittee of the Quality Management Committee. Academy of Nutrition and Dietetics." *J Acad Nutr Diet* 113, 6 suppl (2013): S11–S16.
4. See Note 3 with page numbers: S17–S28.
5. See Note 3 with page numbers: S46–S55.
6. Academy Scope of Practice Decision Tool: A Self-Assessment Guide. "Academy Quality Management Committee and Scope of Practice Subcommittee." *J Acad Nutr Diet* 113, 6 suppl (2013): S10.
7. Academy of Nutrition and Dietetics: Revised 2012 Standards of Practice in Nutrition Care and Standards of Professional Performance for Registered Dietitians. "Academy Quality Management Committee and Scope of Practice Subcommittee of the Quality Management Committee." *J Acad Nutr Diet* 113, z96 suppl (2013): S29–S45.
8. Academy of Nutrition and Dietetics: Revised Standards of Practice in Nutrition Care and Standards of Professional Performance for Dietetic Technicians, Registered. "Academy of Quality Management Committee and Scope of Practice Subcommittee of the Quality Management Committee." *J Acad Nutr Diet* 113, 6 suppl (2013): S56–S71.
9. Price, J.A., S. Kent, S.M. McCauley, J. Parekh, C.J. Klein. "Using Academy Standards of Excellence in Nutrition and Dietetics for Organization Self-Assessment and Quality Improvement." *J Acad Nutr Diet* 114, 8 (2014): 1279–1292.
10. Code of Ethics for the Profession of Dietetics. Accessed May 15, 2016, www .eatright.org
11. Grandgenett, R., and D. Derelian. "Ethics in Business Practice." *J Am Diet Assoc* 110, 7 (2010): 1103–1104.

12. Castle, D., and R. DeBusk. "The Electronic Health Record: Genetic Information and Patient Privacy." *J Am Diet Assoc* 118, 8 (2008): 1372–1374.

13. Ventures. Newsletter of Nutrition Entrepreneurs DPG. "Nutrition Blog Network." *Acad Nutr Diet* XXXVII, 1 (2010): 2.

14. Aase, S. "Toward E-Professionalism: Thinking Through the Implications of Navigating the Digital World." *J Am Diet* Assoc 110, 10 (2010): 1440–1449.

15. Nicklas, J.A., W. Karmally, C.E. O'Neil. "Nutrition Professionals are Obligated to Follow Ethical Guidelines when Conducting Industry-Funded Research." *J Am Diet Assoc* 111, 12 (2011): 1931–1932.

16. Academy of Nutrition and Dietetics. "Registered Dietitian Nutritionists and Nutrition and Dietetics Technicians, Registered, Are Ethically Obligated to Maintain Personal Competence in Practice." *J Acad Nutr Diet* 115, 5 (2015): 811–814.

17. Fornari, A. "Approaches to Ethical Decision-Making." *J Acad Nutr Diet* 115, 1 (2015): 119–121.

18. Rogriguez, J.C. "Culturally Competent Dietetics: Increasing Awareness: Improving Care." *J Am Diet Assoc* 110, 5 (2010): 57.

19. Diversity Strengthens our Academy and Profession. "President's Page." *J Acad Nutr Diet* 115, 10 (2015): 1559.

20. Diversity. Accessed October 29, 2015, www.eatright.org/diversity

21. Bergman, E.A. "Building a Brighter Tomorrow: Diversity, Mentoring, and the Future of Dietetics." *J Acad Nutr Diet* 113, Suppl 3 (2013): S5–S47.

22. Brown, D. "Networking Moves Online." *J Am Diet Assoc* 109, 2 (2010): 210–211.

23. Lane, M. "Streaming Soon to a Computer Near You: How Online Video Will Change Media and Maybe Your Practice Forever." *ADA Times* 108, 1 (2008): 20.

24. Switt, J.T. "Drawing Attention to Your Website." *J Am Diet Assoc* 108, 1 (2008): 20.

25. Hoggle, L.B., M.A. Michael, S.M. Houston, E.J. Ayres. "Nutrition Informatics." *J Am Diet Assoc* 108, 1 (2008): 134–139.

26. Yadrick, M.M. "Informatics: A Word We Need to Know." *J Am Diet Assoc* 108, 1 (2008): 134–139.

27. Aase, Y. "Improved Understanding the Promises and Challenges Nutrition Informatics Poses for Dietetics Careers." *J Am Diet Assoc* 110, 12 (2010): 1794–1795.

28. Murphy, W.J. "A New Breed of Evidence and the Tools to Generate It: Introducing ANDHII." *J Acad Nutr Diet* 115, 1 (2015): 19–26.

29. Department of Health and Human Services. "Understanding Health Information Privacy." Accessed February 12, 2015, www.hhs/gov/ocr/privacy/hipaa

30. Hoggle, L.B., M.A. Michael, S.M. Houston, E.J. Ayres. "Electronic Health Record: Where Does Nutrition Fit In?" *J Am Diet Assoc* 106, 10 (2006): 1688–1695.

31. See Note 30.

32. Derelian, D. "Dietetics: Legalities, Ethics, and Eccentricities." *J Am Diet Assoc* 100, 3 (2000): 519–523.

33. Busey, J.C. "Help! I've Just Been Served." *J Am Diet Assoc* 109, 4 (2009): 600–605.

34. Busey, J.C. "Use of the Word Inadequate—A Legal Perspective." *J Am Diet Assoc* 108, 6 (2008): 935–936.

35. Busey, J.C. "Telehealth—Opportunities and Pitfalls." *J Am Diet Assoc* 109, 8 (2008): 1296–1301.
36. Shanklin, C. "Evidence-Based Practice: Practice Based on Evidence—Right?" *ADA Times* 2003, 3: 1,3.
37. Academy of Nutrition and Dietetics. "Evidence-Based Practice." Accessed October 29, 2015, www.eatright.org
38. Straus, S., and R.B. Haynes. "Managing Evidence-Based Knowledge: The Need for Reliable, Relevant and Readable Resources." *CMAJ* 180, 9 (2009): 942–945.

CHAPTER 6

The Dietitian in Clinical Practice

"We need both cognitive ability and emotional intelligence to help people understand and use the Dietary Guidelines."[1]

OUTLINE

- · Summary
- · Definitions
- · References

LEARNING OBJECTIVES

The student will be able to:

1. Become familiar with employment settings for clinical dietitians.
2. Name the members of the clinical team and their functions.
3. Discuss how clinical services may be organized.
4. Understand the range of responsibilities in clinical practice.
5. Gain information about the future outlook in clinical practice.

INTRODUCTION

The discipline of clinical dietetics originated in 1899 when *dietitian* was defined by the American Home Economics Association as "individuals with a knowledge of food who provide diet therapy for the medical profession."[2] Until 1917, dietitians were affiliated with this association, but after 1917 they belonged to the newly formed American Dietetic Association.[3]

The earliest dietitians worked primarily in hospitals or were associated with food-assistance programs. During the 1930s and 1940s, dietitians became involved in either food production and food service or in the planning and provision of diets for special medical needs. The title, *therapeutic dietitian*, was used to describe the person who provided food for medical reasons, such as the prevention of a nutrient deficiency or to help with the treatment of disease.[4] Examples of early diet therapy are the Sippy diet that used milk and cream to treat ulcers and the Kempner rice diet to treat hypertension; each was named for the physician who designed it.

As the dietitian's role in the hospital became one of providing specialized care and modifying diets to treat various medical conditions, the title, *clinical dietitian*, replaced the former titles.

In the early 1970s, reports of widespread malnutrition among hospitalized patients helped to increase the visibility of clinical dietitians.[5] Clinical dietitians began to take a more active role in screening and monitoring patients along with the provision of nutrition support. Development of individual nutrition care plans became important functions of clinical dietitians. As the role of diet in the etiology of chronic diseases became better defined, clinical dietitians began to spend a greater percentage of their time participating in the prevention of diseases, such as heart disease, cancer, and diabetes.

EMPLOYMENT SETTINGS OF DIETITIANS AND DIETETIC TECHNICIANS

In the 2015 survey of registered dietitians (RDs) and dietetic technicians, registered (DTRs), 84 percent of those contacted reported they were currently employed in dietetics.[6] This high percentage of dietitians and dietetic technicians who were working in the field of dietetics reflected the diversity of job opportunities. **Tables 6-1–6-3** show the primary employment areas of dietitians. Fifty-seven percent of RDs and 56 percent of DTRs were employed in clinical areas of practice. These findings and earlier membership surveys with similar findings indicate stability in these employment areas and that clinical of practice are the predominate area chosen area by entry-level professionals.

Table 6-1. Primary Practice Area of Dietitians

	RDs (%)	DTRs (%)
Clinical nutrition—acute care/inpatient	32	42
Clinical nutrition—ambulatory care	17	1
Clinical nutrition—long-term care	8	13
Community nutrition	10	15
Food and nutrition management	11	17
Consultation and business	8	3
Education and research	7	1

Base: 8853 RDs and DTRs.

Reprinted from *Journal of the Academy of Nutrition and Dietetics*, Volume 112, Number 1 (January 2012), Ward. B. "Compensation and Benefits Survey 2011, Moderate Growth in Registered Dietitian and Dietetic Technician, Registered, Compensation in the Past 2 years," 29–40, Copyright 2012, with permission from Elsevier.

Table 6-2. Highest Number of Positions in Clinical Practice—RDs

	RDs (%)
Clinical dietitian	16
Outpatient dietitian, general	5
Outpatient dietitian, specialist—diabetes	3
Outpatient dietitian, specialist—renal	3
Clinical dietitian, long-term care	8
Women, infants, and children nutritionist	5
Director of food and nutrition services	4
Public Health Nutritionist	3

Reproduced from *Ward. B. Compensation and Benefits Survey* 2011, Moderate Growth in Registered Dietitian and Dietetic Technician, Registered, Compensation in the past 2 years. *Acad Nutr Diet J* 2012(112);29-40. Reprinted from Journal of the Academy of Nutrition and Dietetics, Volume 112, Number 1 (January 2012)

The primary areas of clinical practice are as follows:

1. Acute care/inpatient
   a. Hospitals
2. Ambulatory care
   a. Hospital outpatient departments
   b. Clinics
   c. Outpatient care centers
3. Long-term care
   a. Nursing homes
   b. Assisted living facilities
   c. Alzheimer's disease units

Table 6-3. Highest Number of Positions—DTRs

	DTR
Dietetic technician, clinical	41
Dietetic technician, long-term care	12
WIC nutritionists	5
Director of food and nutrition service	5
Food service management	9

Reprinted from *Journal of the Academy of Nutrition and Dietetics*, Volume 112, Number 1 (January 2012), Ward. B. "Compensation and Benefits Survey 2011, Moderate Growth in Registered Dietitian and Dietetic Technician, Registered, Compensation in the Past 2 years," 29–40, Copyright 2012, with permission from Elsevier.

PRACTICE AUDIT ACTIVITIES

The Commission on Dietetic Registration conducts a practice audit every 5 years. The practice areas of RDs and DTRs are compared to show where there is a higher level of involvement. In clinical practice, the particular areas in which RDs indicate a higher level of involvement than DTRs include the following:[7]

- Principles of *education* including designing courses and evaluating education programs.
- Conducting research. Designing, developing proposals, reporting at professional conferences, and writing for publication.
- Providing nutrition care to individuals. This comprised the largest area of activity as would be expected and included development of institutional standards for nutrition care, evaluating clients' overall health status, recommending and writing orders for tube feedings, parenteral nutrition, medications, etc.
- Providing nutrition programs for population groups, which included designing services to meet nutrition-related needs of groups.

The 2015 Entry-Level Dietetics Practice Audit may be accessed at: Rogers D, Griswold K, Leibowitz PK, Sauer KL, Doughten S. Distinctions in Entry-Level Registered Dietitian Nutritionist and Nutrition and Dietetics Technicians, Registered: Further Results from the 2015 Commission on Dietetic Registration Entry-Level Dietetics Practice Audit. J Acad Nutr Diet 116 (2016) No. 10:1685–1696.

ORGANIZATION OF CLINICAL NUTRITION SERVICES

Clinical nutrition services may be organized in several ways, depending on the setting. In most hospitals, clinical nutrition services are managed by the director of clinical nutrition, or the chief clinical dietitian. Typically, the chief clinical dietitian reports to an individual whose primary responsibilities are overall management of the entire food and nutrition department. In others, clinical dietetics may be organized as a separate department that reports to an executive or administrator with other patient care responsibilities such as nursing or pharmacy. There are advantages and disadvantages to both types of organization. Combining clinical nutrition with food services can facilitate communication regarding patient food choices and menus. By contrast, clinical nutrition as a separate department may increase visibility as an important patient care service unit distinct from food service.

RESPONSIBILITIES IN CLINICAL DIETETICS

Nutrition Care Process and Model

The Quality Management Committee of the Academy of Nutrition and Dietetics developed a nutrition care process (NCP) and model that was adopted by the house of delegates of the American Dietetic Association in 2003.[8] The purpose of the planning model was "for implementation and dissemination to the dietetics profession and the association for the enhancement of the practice of dietetics."[9] The NCP is defined as systematic problem-solving methods that dietetic professionals use to critically think and make decisions to address nutrition-related problems and to provide safe and effective quality nutrition care. Several models were developed before adoption of the present model.

In 2008, a review and update of the process was undertaken following a survey of ADA groups experienced in using the NCP.[11] The process, now referred to as the nutrition care process and model (NCPM), included revisions in the original model and defined the functions under each step as follows (**Figure 6-1**):

1. *Nutrition assessment.* In step 1, a systematic approach to collect, record, and interpret relevant data from patients, clients, family members, caregivers, and other individual groups is undertaken. Examples of the type of data collected are food and nutrition-related history, anthropometric measurements, biochemical data, medical tests and procedures, nutrition-focused physical examination findings, and client history.

2. *Nutrition diagnosis.* Nutrition professionals identify and label existing nutrition problems they are responsible for treating independently. The determination for continuation of care follows this step.

3. *Nutrition intervention.* Action is taken with the intent of changing a nutrition-related behavior, risk factor, environmental condition, or aspect of health status. This entails writing a plan of care, collaborating with the patient or client to identify goals of the interaction, and partnering with the patient and other caregivers to carry out the plan.

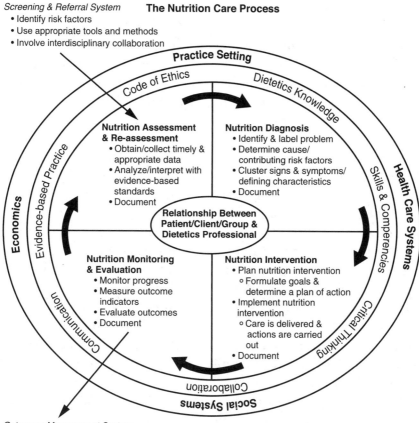

Screening & Referral System   **The Nutrition Care Process**
• Identify risk factors
• Use appropriate tools and methods
• Involve interdisciplinary collaboration

Practice Setting

Code of Ethics   Dietetics Knowledge

Nutrition Assessment & Re-assessment
• Obtain/collect timely & appropriate data
• Analyze/interpret with evidence-based standards
• Document

Nutrition Diagnosis
• Identify & label problem
• Determine cause/contributing risk factors
• Cluster signs & symptoms/defining characteristics
• Document

Relationship Between Patient/Client/Group & Dietetics Professional

Nutrition Monitoring & Evaluation
• Monitor progress
• Measure outcome indicators
• Evaluate outcomes
• Document

Nutrition Intervention
• Plan nutrition intervention
  ○ Formulate goals & determine a plan of action
• Implement nutrition intervention
  ○ Care is delivered & actions are carried out
• Document

Economics   Evidence-based Practice   Communication   Collaboration   Social Systems   Critical Thinking   Skills & Competencies   Health Care Systems

Outcomes Management System
• Monitor the success of the Nutrition Care Process implementation
• Evaluate the impact with aggregate data
• Identify and analyze causes of less than optimal performance and outcomes
• Refine the use of the Nutrition Care Process

FIGURE 6-1. The Nutrition Care Process and Model.

Reprinted from *Journal of the American Dietetic Association* 108, no. 7 (July 2008), "Nutrition Care Process and Model," 1116, 2008, with permission from Elsevier.

4. *Nutrition monitoring and evaluation*. In this final step, the amount of progress is identified and whether the goals and expected outcomes are being met is determined. Three steps are involved, which are as follows:
   a. Monitor progress.
   b. Measure the outcomes.
   c. Evaluate the outcomes by comparing to earlier status or reference standards.

A standardized set of terms has been developed to describe the results in each step of the NCPM.[12] The terms help facilitate the inclusion of RD activities in electronic health record keeping, and also in policies, procedures, rules, and legislation. The use of such standardized reporting primarily assists in documenting nutrition care in the medical record in a way that will refer to each of the four steps in the NCPM and highlight the role of nutrition in patient care.

Medical Nutrition Therapy

Medical nutrition therapy (MNT) has been defined as "all diagnostic, therapeutic, or counseling services provided by an RD for management or treatment of any disease, condition, disorder, or illness."[13] A history of the development of MNT, its importance in the national healthcare discussion, and the challenges presented to members were discussed by the government relations office of the ADA in 2005.[14] Established by legislation under Medicare Part B, provision was made for Medicare reimbursement to dietitians for care in two disease conditions—diabetes and renal disease. The stipulation was that Medicare MNT providers must use evidence-based protocols or guides for practice to illustrate that the MNT offered by RDs has a positive medical impact on patients and a positive impact on healthcare budgets. The rationale and justification for the successful passage of legislation extending MNT to other disease treatments depends, in large part, on the evidence that can be demonstrated regarding its beneficial effects. Cost containment is a critical part of all healthcare reform measures, and passage of any new MNT therapies will demand good scientific evidence of both its cost-effectiveness and efficacy. To this end, evidence-based outcomes research that documents the clinical effectiveness of MNT is all important. Evidence-based practice (EBP), it follows, improves the quality of care and helps manage costs. By adopting EBP in providing MNT, RDs will use the best available evidence to provide therapy, in addition to their own clinical expertise and experience.

The academy assists dietitians by maintaining a library of resources, the Evidence Analysis Library (EAL), available online at www .adaevidencelibrary.com. The EAL gathers the best, most current, and most relevant research on important questions in dietetic practice and is available at no cost to all ADA members.[15] The EAL offers evidence-based nutrition practice guidelines in areas such as lipid metabolism, adult weight management, and critical illnesses.

It can be noted that MNT describes the broad area of practice formerly called diet therapy or therapeutic dietetics, and NCPM is the application of nutrition therapies to disease conditions including guides for nutrition education and preventive nutrition care services.

Standards of Practice

The *Standards of Practice* in nutrition care describe the minimum expectations for competent nutrition care practice. The *Standards of Professional Performance* (SOPP), a companion document, describe the expectation for competent behavior in the nondirect patient or client nutrition care aspect of RD and DTR roles. First developed in 2005, the standards were updated in 2008 and again in 2012.[16]

The standards of practice (SOP) in nutrition care specify the following:

- Address activities related to patient/client care during the NCP.
- Apply to RDs and DTRs who have direct contact with individual patient/client care in acute and long-term care as well as in public health, community, extended care, and ambulatory care settings.
- Formatted according to the four steps of the NCP (i.e., nutrition assessment, nutrition diagnosis, nutrition intervention, and nutrition monitoring and evaluation).
- Reflect the individual levels (RD and DTR) of training, responsibility, and accountability.

The SOPP include the following:

- Address behaviors related to the professional role that are not in the NCP.
- Apply to RDs and DTRs in all practice settings.
- Address six domains of professional performance (i.e., provision of services; application of research; communication and application of knowledge; use and management of resources; quality in practice; and competence and accountability).
- Reflect the individual levels (RD and DTR) of training, responsibility, and accountability.

THE CLINICAL NUTRITION SERVICE TEAM

Clinical nutrition services may be provided by a number of team members in healthcare facilities. Inpatient nutritional care in hospitals is usually the responsibility of persons in several positions—clinical nutrition managers or chief clinical dietitians, clinical dietitians, dietetic technicians, and dietetic assistants. Outpatient clinics and ambulatory care centers may use all four positions but are more likely to employ only clinical dietitians. Extended care facilities and physician offices may have clinical dietitians on staff; however, more often these facilities use a consulting dietitian to provide MNT for selected patients and clients. Consulting dietitians may be in private practice or part of a group practice.

Clinical Nutrition Manager or Chief Clinical Dietitian

The clinical nutrition manager or chief clinical dietitian is primarily responsible for directing the activities of clinical dietitians, dietetic technicians, and dietetic assistants. Major tasks performed include developing and managing budgets for the clinical area, hiring clinical nutrition employees, evaluating employee job performance, providing in-service and on-the-job training, reviewing productivity reports, writing job descriptions, scheduling employees, developing policies and procedures, designing performance standards, and developing and implementing goals and objectives for the department. The clinical nutrition manager is also responsible for communicating with the staff of other departments and the administration. Ultimately, the clinical nutrition manager ensures that performance is actually accomplished to achieve the goals and objectives for the department. The Clinical Nutrition Management dietetic practice group provides a newsletter and a yearly workshop on practice updates and opportunities for networking with peers.

Clinical Dietitian

The primary responsibility of the clinical dietitian is to provide nutritional care for patients. Clinical dietitians in hospitals are involved in nutritional screening for patients to determine the presence of or risk of developing malnutrition, to perform nutritional assessments, and to develop nutrition care plans. Clinical nutrition services may be provided to general patient-care units or may be based on a medical specialization (e.g., critical care or diabetes education). Clinical dietitians are important members of the healthcare team because they consult and collaborate with physicians, pharmacists, nurses, social workers, chaplains, and others in providing nutritional care.

Clinical dietitians are the source of authoritative knowledge about MNT and patient nutrition education. They routinely communicate with other disciplines regarding developments in MNT and patient education through in-service teams, rounds, and multidisciplinary patient care conferences.

Successful clinical dietitians in acute healthcare facilities must also be able to apply managerial concepts to provide effective nutritional care. Management tasks often performed by clinical dietitians include scheduling of patient care services, in-service training, on-the-job training, employee interviews and evaluations, writing, job descriptions, planning cycle menus, and evaluating the quality of patient food.

Typical activities of a clinical dietitian include the following:[17]

- Use the NCP to screen, assess, diagnose, interview, and evaluate nutritional care of patients.
- Provide instruction to patients and families on nutritional needs.
- Review medical records for information including nutrition-related data.
- Calculate nutrient and fluid requirements.
- Evaluate nutrient intake and make adjustments accordingly.
- Adapt regular diets to meet individual needs or preferences.
- Plan oral diets with multiple nutritional requirements.
- Refer clients to community resources for ongoing service (Women, Infants, and Children program; Mobile Meals, outpatient clinics, and wellness centers).
- Use evidence analysis in making practical decisions about needed care.
- Perform quality assurance and make performance improvements as needed.
- Utilize technology as freely as possible.
- Communicate with physicians, nurses, and other staff.
- Attend medical rounds.
- Provide ongoing evaluation for employees.
- Utilize SOP and SOPP in providing care.
- Serve as preceptor for dietetic interns and other students.

Clinical dietitians may be members of one or more dietetic practice groups. Besides working in general clinical practice, dietitians may be titled gerontological nutritionists, dietitians in developmental and psychiatric disorders, oncology dietitians, renal dietitians, pediatric dietitians, diabetes care and support, dietitians in nutrition support, perinatal nutritionists, and others. The diversity of specialty and subspecialty areas of practice reflects the broad range of interests and opportunities open to the clinical dietitian.

Dietetic Technician

The dietetic technician in the clinical setting assists the clinical dietitian and is a valuable member of the nutrition care team. Typically, major functions performed include gathering data for nutritional screening and assigning a level of risk for malnutrition according to predetermined criteria. He or she may help with nutritional assessments by gathering laboratory and anthropometric data, collecting and analyzing nutritional intakes, obtaining nutritional histories, and reviewing medical histories. Dietetic technicians may administer nourishment and dietary supplements for patients and monitor and document intakes. They may provide information to help patients select menus and give simple diet instructions. Dietetic technicians maintain a high level of knowledge of nutritional care. Management responsibilities of dietetic technicians may also include supervision of dietetic assistants and students.

Dietetic Assistant

The dietetic assistant helps the clinical dietitian and dietetic technician in some of the routine aspects of nutritional care. He or she is often responsible for processing diet orders, checking patient intakes, giving nourishments, and transmitting special food requests. Dietetic assistants may also help distribute and pick up inpatient menus and pass and collect trays. They may be involved in evaluating food acceptance and gathering food records to evaluate and document nutrient intakes.

CLINICAL DIETETICS OUTLOOK

Communicating Nutrition Messages

Dietitians increasingly use technology to both gain and transmit information to clients and the public. They are well qualified to also evaluate information from all sources including the extensive array of material offered on the Internet.[20] Through nutrition Informatics, all dietitians, whether in early learning stages or already proficient in data management, have access to apps and websites for assistance. Nutrition informatics is defined as the "the effective retrieval, organization, storage and optimal use information, data and knowledge for food, and nutrition-related problem solving and decision making."[21] The Academy Nutrition Informatics Committee defines it simply as "the interaction of information, nutrition and technology."[22]

The Informatics committee conducted a Delphi Study in 2011 that resulted in descriptions of five levels of competency in the application of computer skills.[23] They ranged from possessing computer usage skill to becoming an Informatics expert involved in research and work with other health care providers to develop new methods for data and information management.

Technology provides a way to engage patients and clients, to expand the reach of practice and potentially lower health care costs. Through the use of the many apps now available on the Internet, dietitians have many resources to assist in providing information as well as help in sorting through the best and most reliable information. The Nutrition Entrepreneurs DPG and the Clinical Nutrition Managers both have subgroups on technology and informatics.[24] Further, the Informatics Committee began a series in 2015 to introduce different ways practitioners may identify as a "Nutrition Informatics Registered Dietitian."[25]

Dietitians can also take advantage of online courses by long distance offered as "Massive Open Online Courses." They are courses of broad appeal developed by education and other experts that are offered free of charge.[26] They offer a variety of courses in many subject areas including food, nutrition, health, management, and many others.

Electronic Health Records

The passage of the Health Information Technology for Economic and Clinical Health (HITECH) act in 2009 provided for primary physicians and small hospital to adopt electronic health records. Although NRDs or DTRs were not specifically included in the incentives offered, a committee of the Academy is developing ways dietitians can also participate and indeed will need to as the changeover is undertaken by hospitals. An example is information for incorporating Nutrition Care Plan terminology into the system. Dietitians will need to be ready to contribute to the health record as the change from paper records is adopted by 2017.[27]

Clinical Privileging

RDs are now permitted to order patient diets independently without requiring the supervision or approval of a physician or other practitioner. Clinical privileging refers to a process by which a hospital, specifically the governing body and the medical staff of the hospital, develop and implement procedures to ensure safe and quality patient care.[18,19] The approval for this change came in 2014 when the Centers for Medicare and Medicaid published a rule to this effect.[28] The RDN must be privileged to order diets by the hospital in which he or she is employed and comply with any licensing regulations. As well as writing the diet order, the RDN may order lab tests and make modifications to the diet order based on the lab tests. This is a change the Academy has worked toward for a long time and it positions the dietitian as the expert in the patient's nutritional care.

Trends in Clinical Dietetics

Demographic trends have an impact on dietetic practice. For instance, the aging population and especially the growth of the "oldest old" means that nutrition is critical in helping keep this group healthy as long as possible. This is also the group that is at highest risk for chronic diseases that are treated in part with medical nutrition therapy. Increasing diversity among groups served also has implications for dietitians in creating cultural competency and raising awareness.[24]

The obesity/overweight epidemic today is an area in which nutrition education for the public is more important than ever. Dietitians may find increasing opportunities to work with food processors, grocery stores, and advertisers to reach the public with the most effective nutrition messages. All these areas are discussed in more detail later in this text.

SUMMARY

Clinical dietetics is the largest area of employment for dietitians, especially at the entry level. Future roles will expand as new skills and competencies through advanced training and education are attained. Employment opportunities exist in acute care centers, in community-based programs, in consultation and private practice, in communications, and in many entrepreneurial undertakings.

The clinical dietitian is central in helping persons during illness through nutrition interventions. Equally important is helping individuals prevent the onset of chronic disease by the application of optimal nutrition practices throughout life. The expansion of MNT with cost-effectiveness data and demonstration of quality practice is a continuing challenge for the dietetics profession. Even though employment increasingly moves outside the traditional hospital or clinic, the services provided by the clinical dietitians will remain vital to the health and well-being of people experiencing illness and who need nutritional care.

DEFINITIONS

Clinical dietetics. The area of practice in which persons with illness or injury involving nutritional factors are treated using assessment, planning, and implementing nutrition care plans.

Clinical nutrition services. Activities provided in the practice of clinical dietetics, such as medical nutrition therapy and counseling.

Diet therapy. Treatment by diet; a term now replaced by *clinical nutrition therapy* or *medical nutrition therapy.*

Extended care facility. An institution that extends health care beyond the acute care setting when long-term term care is needed.

Medical nutrition therapy. The application of nutrition in the management of illness or injury.

Outpatient clinic. Treatment area of a hospital or healthcare facility in which patients are treated on an outpatient basis.

REFERENCES

1. Escott-Stump, S.A. "Our Nutrition Literacy Challenge: Making the 2010 Dietary Guidelines Relevant for Consumers." *J Acad Nutr Diet* 111 (2011): 979.
2. Cooper, L.F. "The Dietitian and Her Profession." *J Am Diet Assoc* 14 (1938): 751–758.
3. See Note 2, p.752.
4. Huyck, L., and M.M. Rowe. *Managing Clinical Nutrition Services.* (Rockville, MD: Aspen Publisher, 1990), pp. 243.
5. Butterworth, E. "The Skeleton in the Hospital Closet." *Nutrition Today* 4 (1974): 4.
6. Rogers, D. "Compensation and Benefits Survey 2015." *J Acad Nutr Diet* 115, 3 (2015): 370–388.
7. Ward, B.D., D. Rogers, M.M. Mueller, C.R. Touger-Decker, K.L. Sauer, and D. Schmidt. "Distinguishing Entry-Level RD and DTR Practice: Results from the 2010 Commission on Dietetic Registration Entry-Level Dietetics Practice Audit." *J Am Diet Assoc* 111 (2011): 1749–1755.

8. Lacy, K., and E. Pritchett. "Nutrition Care Process and Model: ADA Adopts Road Map to Quality Care and Outcomes Management." *J Am Diet Assoc* 103 (2003): 1061–1071.

9. See Note 8.

10. Hammond, M.L. "Nutrition Care Process and Model: And Academic and Practice Odyssey." *J Acad Nutr Diet* 114, 12 (2014): 1879–1894.

11. Writing Group of the Nutrition Care Process/Standardized Language Committee. *J Am Diet Assoc* 108 (2008): 1113–1117.

12. Writing Group of the Nutrition Care Process and Standardized Language Committee. "Nutrition Care Process and Model Part II: Using the International Dietetics and Nutrition Terminology to Document the Nutrition Care Process." *J Am Diet Assoc* 108 (2008): 1287–1293.

13. Smith, R.E., S. Patrick, P. Michael, and M. Hager. "Medical Nutrition Therapy: The Case of ADA's Advocacy Efforts (Part 1)." *J Am Diet Assoc* 105 (2005): 825–834.

14. Smith, R.E., S. Patrick, P. Michael, and M. Hager. "Medical Nutrition Therapy: The Case of ADA's Advocacy Efforts. (Part II)." *J Am Diet Assoc* 105 (2005): 987–996.

15. Blumberg-Kason, S., and R. Lipscomb. "Evidence-Based Nutrition Practice Guidelines: A Valuable Resource in the Evidence-Analysis Library." *J Am Diet Assoc* 106 (2006): 1935–1936.

16. Boucher, J., A. Evert, A. Daly, K. Kulkami, J.A. Rizzotta, K. Burton, and B. Bradshaw. "American Dietetic Association Revised Standards and Standards of Professional Performance for Registered Dieticians (Generalist, Specialty, and Advanced) in Diabetes Care."

17. Ward, B., C. Mueller, R. Touger-Decker, and K.L. Sauer. "Entry-Level Dietetics Practice Today: Results from the 2010 Commission on Dietetic Registration Entry-Level Dietetics Practice Audit." *J Am Diet Assoc* 111 (2011): 914–941.

18. Hager, M.H. "Clinical Privileging for Registered Dietitians. A Regulatory Perspective." *J Am Diet Assoc* 107 (2007): 558–560.

19. Hager, M.H., and S.M. McCauley. "Clinical Privileging: What It Is—and Isn't." *J Am Diet Assoc* 109 (2009): 400–402.

20. Communicating Accurate Food and Nutrition Information. "Practice Paper by the Academy of Nutrition and Dietetics." *J Acad Nutr Diet* 112, 5 (2012): 759.

21. Ayres, E.J., J.L. Greer-Carney, P.E.F. McShane, A. Miller, and P. Turner. "Nutrition Informatics Competencies across all Level of Practice: A National Delphi Study." *J Acad Nutr Diet* 112, 12 (2012): 2042–2053.

22. See Note 2.

23. Boyce, B. "Nutrition Apps: Opportunities to Guide Patients and Grow Your Career." *J Acad Nutr Diet* 114, 1 (2014): 13–15.

24. Accessed April 11, 2015, www.eatrightPRO.org

25. Stark, C.M. "Massive Open Online Courses: How Registered Dietitians Use MOOCs for Nutrition Education." *J Acad Nutr Diet* 114, 8 (2014): 1147–1155.

26. Accessed May 11, 2015, NCP@eatright.org

27. Accessed March 11, 2015, www.eatrightPRO.org

CHAPTER 7

Management in Food and Nutrition Systems

"Food management RDs need to have technical expertise, knowledge, and interpersonal skills."[1]

OUTLINE

INTRODUCTION

Food and food service are prominent in the history of the profession of dietetics. One of the main purposes of the first organized meeting of the American Dietetic Association (ADA) was to discuss ways of meeting food shortages during World War I. Many of the first members of the association served overseas feeding hospitalized soldiers and people living under wartime conditions. Cooking schools, scientists who produced the first tables of food values, early-day soup kitchens, and school lunch programs were among the forerunners of institutions that fed the public.[2]

Food service in hospitals was the primary focus of the first dietitians. During the 1890s, food service in hospitals was managed by the chef, the housekeeper, or the nursing department. In the early 1900s, however, many dietitians were in charge of dietary departments and had the responsibility for all food service as well as teaching nurses and providing diet therapy for patients with metabolic diseases. Hospital dietitians dealt with budgets, department organization, personnel management, and quality food service. Nutrition was recognized as an aspect of medicine, and food prescriptions were handled as apothecary compounds, thus creating a demand for special diet kitchens. The hospital dietitian had the same status as the superintendent of nurses and was recognized as the nutrition expert.[3]

Dietitians with food service management responsibilities became members of the Food Administration section in the ADA, and their practice was referred to as *administrative dietetics*. The terminology now used is *management in food and nutrition systems*.

Management is discussed fully later in the text as a skill needed by dietitians in all areas of practice.

ACTIVITIES OF ENTRY-LEVEL DIETITIANS AND DIETETIC TECHNICIANS

In 2010, the Commission on Dietetic Registration conducted a practice audit among dietitians and dietetic technicians and indicated the percentage of time spent in selected activities. Management activities of both groups are shown in **Table 7-1**.

Table 7-1.   Management Activities of Entry-Level Dietitians and Dietetic Technicians

Activity (Percent)	RD	DTR[a]
Managing human resources		
Assign or schedule staff	15	25
Male decisions on personnel actions	10	23
Comply with labor relations	15	23
Evaluate performance of staff	22	31
Managing food and material resources		
Maintain safety and sanitation of food, facilities, or equipment	27	53
Monitor stage conditions	22	39
Develop menus for clients with normal needs	33	45
Evaluate food products by taste, smell, and appearance	33	50
Calculate quantities to purchase of food other material resources	9	21
Purchase food, nutritional supplements, equipment, or supplies	14	24
Assess client satisfaction with food and/or nutrition service	40	59
Adjust daily menu, food production, or distribution based on availability of food, labor, or equipment	11	30
Institute or maintain sustainability practices	8	18

(continues)

Table 7-1.   Management Activities of Entry-Level Dietitians and Dietetic Technicians (Continued)

Activity (Percent)	RD	DTRª
Manage facilities		
Maintain facilities and equipment	11	24
Assure safety of employees, patients, clients, and customers	25	38

a. The higher percentages of involvement by dietetic technicians in many of the management categories reflect the areas in which technicians are most often employed. This was a survey of entry-level professionals, and it should be noted that more dietitians begin their careers in clinical areas of practice; this was borne out in those particular areas surveyed.

Notes: RD 5 registered dietitian; DTR 5 dietetic technician, registered.

Reprinted from *Journal of the American Dietetic Association* 111, Number 11 (November 2011), Ward, B., D. Rogers, C. Mueller, R. Touger-Decker, KI.L. Sauer, C. Schmidt, "Distinguishing Entry-Level RD and DTR Practice: Results from the 2010 Commission on Dietetic Registration Entry-Level Dietetics Practice Audit, 1749–1755," Copyright 2011, with permission from Elsevier.

AREAS OF EMPLOYMENT

In the 2015 membership survey, 11 percent of registered dietitians (RDs) and 17 percent of dietetic technicians, registered (DTRs) indicated their practice is in food and nutrition management. Further, 24 percent of practitioners are executives, directors, or managers, and another 17 percent are supervisors or coordinators.[4]

In the same study, it was reported that salaries for the food and nutrition manager are the highest of those in any practice area. The salaries reflect both geographic location and years of experience as the food and nutrition manager is nearly always a dietitian with work experience beyond entry level and may have an advanced degree or a business degree.

Dietitians in food and nutrition management typically affiliate with one or more of the following five dietetic practice groups: Management in Food and Nutrition Systems, Dietitians in Business and Communication, School Nutrition Services, Food and Culinary Professionals, and Hunger and Environmental Nutrition. In addition, clinical managers may belong to the Clinical Nutrition Management group. Dietitians in food and nutrition management may be identified through a wide range of titles, such as coordinator, specialist, executive dietitian, director of food and nutrition services, director of clinical nutrition, or chief administrator.

Practice areas are often categorized by work settings, such as food and nutrition management in acute care, long-term care, and noninstitutional employment areas. To encompass the broader management area, clinical nutrition management, commercial food service, and school nutrition are added to this list. A discussion of each follows.

Food and Nutrition Management in Acute Care

Food service in acute care is the type of service provided in hospitals or similar healthcare institutions in which patients receive short-term medical treatment, usually 1–5 days. Several characteristics of this type of food service are:

1. Fast turnover of patients with day-to-day fluctuations in the number of meals prepared and served.
2. Special diets requiring different types of food preparation. In some instances, as many as 50 percent of all patients will require special or modified diets.
3. Selective menus for patients, increasing the number of food items prepared.
4. Multiple serving systems in an institution, such as individual tray service, decentralized service with pantries on patient floors, and restaurant-style service providing individualized patient service.

In some institutions, food is prepared in bulk, then preportioned and held until the time of meal service, when it is rethermalized and served. In others, food is prepared centrally just before meal service and either portioned individually or sent in bulk to patient areas for individual service. Production and food service systems vary, but in each system, the dietitian has overall responsibility for food production and service or may share this responsibility with a dietetic technician, chef, or manager. Whatever the scope of his or her responsibility, the dietitian must be knowledgeable in food production techniques, food purchasing, safety and sanitation, strategic planning, human relations, communication skills, managerial skills, and financial management.

Food and Nutrition Management in Long-Term Care Facilities

The provision of food for clients in nursing homes, extended care facilities, and correctional institutions is included in the long-term care category. Food service in these institutions differs from that in acute care in that clients are long term and are usually served in group settings. Central food production and few special diets are typical because most of the long-term clients will be following a normal, healthy eating pattern. The food service, especially in smaller nursing homes and extended care facilities, may be managed by a dietetic technician or by a certified dietary manager under the direction of a dietitian consultant. In correctional institutions, the day-to-day management is often provided by nonprofessionals under the direction of a dietitian consultant when one is available. All aspects of food service management are equally as important in long-term care as in the hospital with the added necessity of ensuring nutritional adequacy and acceptability over longer periods of time. In almost all long-term facilities, there are federal and state regulations relating to the provision of food services to clients that must be followed for the institution to receive government funding and provide quality care. The qualifications for the food service manager are also specified in the regulations.

Food and Nutrition Management in Noninstitutional Settings

Management of food and nutrition in noninstitutional settings is typically provided in colleges and universities, employee cafeterias, and business and commercial enterprises. The food service may be for-profit or nonprofit, depending on the type of institution. Generally, institutions serving the public will be for profit while schools or businesses providing employee food services are more often nonprofit. Clients choose to patronize the food services offered and the type of food services may vary widely. A college or university, for instance, may offer cafeteria, dining room, restaurant, catering, and vending services. School and employee food service is often provided by cafeteria service along with vending and dining room service. Many businesses provide employee cafeterias or restaurant service. The dietitian's responsibility is to provide food that is safe and acceptable to the customers, meets financial expectations, and promotes good nutrition.

School Nutrition Programs

School nutrition programs, offering either lunch or breakfast, or both, are available in 100,000 public schools through grade 12, nonprofit private schools, and residential child care institutions.[5] Over 31 million students from preschool through grade 12 were fed daily. An average of 11 million children per day participated in the federal school breakfast program in

2009. The programs are administered and partially funded by the federal government, and they must meet specific guidelines for nutritional quality of meals and for student eligibility. Free or reduced-price meals are provided based on the family economic status. The emphasis is on long-term health benefits for children through establishing good eating habits. The following is a position statement supporting school nutrition programs:

> It is the position of the Academy, School Nutrition Association, and Society for Nutrition Education that comprehensive, integrated nutrition services in schools, kindergarten through grade 12, are an essential component of coordinated school health programs that will improve the nutritional status, health, and academic performance of our nation's children. Local school wellness policies may strengthen comprehensive nutrition services in schools by providing opportunities for multidisciplinary teams to identify and address local school needs.[6]

Dietitians in school nutrition programs need both managerial and nutrition education skills. That school nutrition programs provide satisfying careers to many is shown in a recent study of job satisfaction; dietitians with management responsibilities, including those in school child nutrition programs, showed the highest level of satisfaction with the nature of the work and a higher overall level of satisfaction compared to national indices.[7]

The customer is the most important consideration when offering school food service that meets strict guidelines for safety and nutritional quality while also controlling costs.[8] Some programs use websites to promote offerings and others use newspaper advertising to publish menus and gain public support.

Clinical Nutrition Management

As discussed earlier, the clinical nutrition manager is the professional who directs the activities of a clinical unit in hospitals and healthcare institutions. This may include responsibility for one or more units and the supervision of other professionals in clinical areas. The clinical manager performs many of the same management functions as the food service dietitian—management of human, financial, and material resources. The clinical dietitian who progresses from an entry-level position to a management position will normally have 5–10 years or more of experience and may not be involved in day-to-day activities directly related to patient care.

Commercial Food Service

Commercial food service is described as retail and hospitality food service establishments that prepare food for immediate consumption on or off premises. The types of establishments employing dietitians include independent restaurants, catering services, casual and family dining restaurants, and fine dining restaurants. Supermarket chains, limited service (fast-food) chains, and hotel chains also have high potential for dietetic services. Five specific areas of need in these institutions are nutrition education, healthful menu planning, recipe and menu analysis, marketing, and quality assurance.

Skills in public relations, communications, marketing, purchasing, and financial management are expected of dietitians who work in commercial food services. Therefore, additional training and experience are often needed by the dietitian to be fully qualified for these roles.

Additional Areas of Opportunity

Additional opportunities for dietitians in food service management include positions in food corporations, such as research and development, consumer affairs, communications, government liaison, emergency feeding for displaced persons, disaster planning centers, military-based homeless shelters and food distribution centers, worldwide religious ministries and government food programs, adult and child care programs, and academic units with food, nutrition, or hospitality programs. Many dietitians are employed in contract food service companies that provide for-profit management services. Hospitals, colleges and universities, schools, employee cafeterias in businesses, hotels and restaurants, and healthcare institutions may contract with a company who manages food services for a negotiated fee. The companies hire and often train their own personnel, including dietitian managers.

CHARACTERISTICS OF SUCCESSFUL FOOD AND NUTRITION MANAGERS

Employment areas in food and nutrition management require registered dietitian nutritionist (RDN) leaders who are effective in the management of human, material, and financial resources. Food and nutrition services in healthcare facilities are becoming more complex in meeting the demands of the administration, patients, and clients. From a historical standpoint, meal service to patients was the primary focus of foodservice departments in healthcare especially in hospitals. Services are now expected in other units within an institution as shown in **Figure 7-1**.

With this expansion of services offered, the RDN and DTR have a wide scope of practice responsibilities in healthcare systems as well as in business, industry, and consulting. These include planning, organizing, staffing, budgeting, directing, and controlling.[9] Managers must make decisions in the best interests of both the department and the institution and be able to communicate effectiveness to the organization's leadership. The productivity of the department is directly related to the quality of the managerial decisions and to the outcomes of departmental efforts.

According to Puckett,[9] today's management RDN must, at a minimum, possess competencies in the following areas:

- Environmental protection rules
- The political environment
- Marketing and customer satisfaction
- Continual quality improvement
- Work design and productivity
- Innovative cost-containment measures
- Food consumption patterns
- Human resource trends
- Food and water safety
- Disaster and emergency planning
- Project and process management
- Cultural diversity in the marketplace

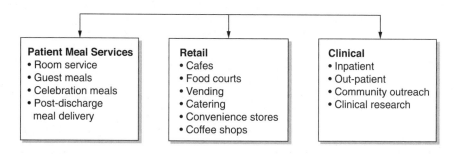

FIGURE 7-1. Scope of Services.

Reproduced from Practice Paper of the Academy of Nutrition and Dietetics: Principles of Productivity in Food and Nutrition Services: Applications in the 21st Century Health Care Reform Era. *J Acad Nutr Diet* 2015;115(7):1141–1147.

Competencies typical of visionary leaders who are effective in their position and in the organization and who are successful in their practice are shown in **Table 7-2.**

As in other areas of practice, the RDN in food service management usually begins at a *competent* level of knowledge and skills at entry-level following registration. The next stage is *proficiency* in operational skills and the possible beginning of specialist credentials followed by the *expert* who continues to build on his/her knowledge, skills, and credentials.[10]

Table 7-2. Competencies Needed by Healthcare Food Service Managers

Successful healthcare food service managers will:

- Use management techniques to cultivate relationships in and out of the institution and achieve cooperation through teamwork.
- Demonstrate effective communications to achieve understanding of personnel and departmental policies.
- Achieve an organizational structure, mission statement, policies, and procedures that effect necessary changes when indicated.
- Possess technological knowledge of food service, practice experience, and external business and administrative needs.
- Use management techniques based on sound character, compassion, insight, and personal integrity.
- Exhibit personal behaviors and attitudes consistent with professional and institutional goals.
- Pursue professional knowledge and growth.
- Possess effective supervisory and managerial skills to derive optimal employee performance.
- Achieve ways to enhance performance and growth of employee.
- Understand the policies of the institution and an ability to interface effectively with superiors.
- Exhibit effective use of resource (fiscal, personnel, and material) to facilitate planning and current operations.
- Possess analytic and decision-making techniques to achieve maximum quality for customer and clients.
- Formulate a creative vision that integrates mutually satisfying department and institutional goals.

Adapted from *Journal of the American Dietetic Association*, 95, Watabe-Dawson, M. "Visionary Leaders Are Key to Success in Food Service," p. 13. Copyright 1995, with permission from Elsevier.

EXPANDED OPPORTUNITIES

Entry-level dietitians with management responsibilities are employed primarily in food service or clinical nutrition service operations. The predominant responsibilities at this level involve technical skills that ensure that food is procured, managed, prepared, and delivered to patients and other clients, and that appropriate nutrition services are provided. With experience and perhaps advanced study, conceptual skills are utilized to identify problem areas requiring attention, to select appropriate techniques, analyze alternative strategies, and select solutions consistent with organization goals.

From entry-level positions, dietitians may advance to the assistant or associate director level of a department and eventually to director or chief administrator. They may manage multidepartmental units or a complex of smaller hospitals, specialty clinics, or long-term care centers. They may become the chief operating officer of a healthcare facility.

Dietitians directing food and nutrition services must have a diversified, multipurpose, broad-based education and experiences from which to draw for expanded roles. They must be familiar with applicable computer software, business organization, marketing, labor relations, industrial engineering, writing and media relations, public relations, financial management data evaluation, policy formation and problem solving, decision making, negotiation, behavior modification techniques, and dealing with challenges.

EXPANSION OF ROLES

Expanded roles may include new and challenging positions that come from the foundation the dietitian receives and that may not even generally be associated with dietetics. In health care, for instance, there is heightened consumer interest in what constitutes healthy food. The food industry wants effective marketing of its products, including information about safety and nutrient value, and wants to develop new products. All these areas represent opportunities in consumer education, writing, food safety, media positions, public policy, food demonstration, and more.

Disaster planning and emergency training is a further need for the food service manager. In events such as floods, hurricanes, earthquakes, and fires, the availability of food and water becomes of paramount concern.[11] "Nutrition security," defined as "secure access to appropriate diets, a sanitary environment and adequate health services and care," may become huge issues if they are not met.[12] Fortunately there are many evidence-based food-related resources available to RDNs and DTRs for personal training and to share with clients and others in public health and healthcare settings. The Food and Drug Administration, the Centers for Disease Control and Prevention, organizations, and the Internet all provide resource materials. The U.S. Department of Agriculture also maintains a hot line for food safety information.[12] A tutorial on disaster planning is available from the Academy.[13] Many local, state, and national groups provide credible sources of information and training in these areas. The RDN or DTR may also consider obtaining certificates of training offered by groups such as the Food Marketing Institute, the National Restaurant Association, the National Registry of Food Safety Professionals, and others. Such certifications can be further used to meet requirements for professional development and to maintain state licensure credentials.[14]

Interesting and informative accounts of events during actual world disasters such as the Japanese earthquake and Hurricane Sandy in New Orleans give insight into how food and nutrition issues can be handled.[15,16]

A new dimension in foodservice management is the use of automation to simplify many tasks—especially those of a repetitive or dangerous nature. With the rapid advances in technology today, machines may take over many foodservice tasks in the future. An example of one type of automation under development is an optical scanner that analyzes food for nutrient content, actual ingredients, and any additives or contaminants.[17] A database of standard foods and food varieties is to be developed after which it will be possible to test whether the food contains what the label claims and allowing reliable and immediate information to the manager.

Machines could conceivably take over tasks such as cleaning, trash collecting, controlling temperatures, tray delivery and pickup, managing storerooms, loading and unloading dish machines, and others. The foodservice manager needs to be cognizant of emerging technological trends such as these in order to make decisions about their applicability in practice.[18]

SUMMARY

The dietitian in food service management has career opportunities in food, food production and service, management, and the higher levels of activities associated with management and leadership. For the motivated and skilled dietitians, higher salary levels and greater degrees of responsibility and self-actualization can be realized.

DEFINITIONS

Food production. The process of preparing and serving food, including purchasing, storage, and processing.

Food services. Production and service of food; also refers to the unit or group responsible for feeding groups.

Food service systems. Activities that together form the inputs, transformation, and outputs that make up an entire food operation.

Human resources. The personnel in an organization.

Management. The administration and coordination of the activities and functions in an organizational unit.

Quality assurance. The certification of the continual, optimal, effective, and efficient outcomes of a service or program.

Resource allocation. The equitable distribution of financial, physical, and human capital.

REFERENCES

1. Puckett, R.P., W. Barkley, G. Dixon, K. Egan, C. Koch, T. Malone, J. Scott-Smith, B. Sheridan, et al. "The American Dietetic Association Standards of Professional Performance for Registered Dietitians (Generalist and Advanced) in Management of Food and Nutrition Systems." *J Am Diet Assoc* 109 (2009): 540–543.
2. Cassell, J.A. *Carry the Flame: The History of the American Dietetic Association.* (Chicago: American Dietetic Association, 1990).
3. Barker, A., M. Foltz, M.B.F. Arensberg, and M.R. Schiller. *Leadership in Dietetics: Achieving a Vision for the Future.* (Chicago: American Dietetic Association, 1994).
4. Rogers, D. "Compensation and Benefits Survey 2015." *J Acad Nutr Diet* 115, no. 3 (2015): 370–388.

5. www.fns.usda/gov/nslp/national (3/20/16).

6. "Position of the American Dietetic Association, School Nutrition Association, and Society for Nutrition Education: Comprehensive School Nutrition Services." *J Acad Nutr Diet* 110 (2010): 1738–1748.

7. Sauer, K., D. Canter, and C. Shanklin. "Job Satisfaction of Dietitians with Management Responsibilities: An Exploratory Study Supporting ADA's Research Priorities." *J Am Diet Assoc* 110 (2010): 1432–1440.

8. Boyce, B. "Satisfying Customers and Lowering Costs in Foodservice: Can Both Be Accomplished Simultaneously?" *J Acad Nutr Diet* 111 (2011): 1458–1466.

9. Puckett, R.P. "Leadership Managing for Change." In *Food Service Manual for Health Care Institutions*, 3rd ed. (San Francisco: Jossey-Bass, 2004), p. 30–32.

10. Berthelsen, R.M., W.C. Barclay, P.M. Oliver, V. McLymont, R. Puckett. "Academy of Nutrition and Dietetics: Revised 2014 Standards of Professional Performance for Registered Nutritionist in Management of Food and Nutrition Systems." *J Acad Nutr Diet* 114, no. 7 (2014): 1104–1112.

11. "Position of the Academy of Nutrition and Dietetics: Food and Water Safety." *J Acad Nutr Diet* 114, no. 11 (2014): 1819–1828.

12. See Note 11.

13. www.eatright.org/disaster (4/3/15).

14. See Note 11.

15. Amagai, T., S. Ichimaru, M. Tai, Y. Ejira, A. Muto. "Nutrition in the Great East Japan Earthquake Disaster." *Nutr in Clin Pract* 29, no. 5 (2014): 585–594.

16. Trent L, Allen S. "Hurricane Sandy: Nutrition Support During Disasters." *Nutr I Clin Pract* 29, no. 5 (2014): 576–584.

17. Washington Post: March 30, 2016.

18. "Man and Machine Knowledge Work in the Age of the Algorithm." *Harvard Business Review* (June 2015): 57–65.

CHAPTER 8

The Public Health/ Community Nutrition Dietitian

"Primary prevention is the most effective and affordable course of action for preventing and reducing the risk for chronic disease."[1]

OUTLINE

LEARNING OBJECTIVES

The student will be able to:
1. Describe Public Health Nutrition and Community Nutrition Practice.
2. Become familiar with the activities of the community dietitian in community settings and programs.

3. Understand the role of nutritionists in public health and ways they may differ from the traditional community nutrition setting.
4. Relate how public health programs promote the prevention of disease.
5. Become aware of specialty areas of practice in community nutrition.

INTRODUCTION

Public health/community nutrition is an area of nutrition and dietetics practice that addresses the entire range of food and nutrition issues relating to individuals, families, and special groups with a common bond such as place of work, place of residence, language, culture, and health. Community nutrition programs include those that provide increased access to food, food and nutrition, and health care. Public health is the component of community nutrition that is publicly funded and provided through a state or local health agency to promote health, prevent disease, and provide primary care. The "community dietitian," "community nutritionist," or "public health nutritionist" provides nutrition services to identified groups.

Professionals in this area of practice establish links with other professionals involved in a broad range of human services, including child care agencies, services for the elderly, churches, summer feeding programs, educational institutions, and researchers. They focus on promoting optimum health and preventing disease in the community by using a population focus and a client or personal health service approach.

Community nutrition is influenced by the collective beliefs and practices of everyone in the community. For instance, it is estimated that about 70 percent of all premature deaths in the United States are caused by environmental factors and individual behaviors.[2] The costs of health care for obesity and its complications continue to rise as this controllable condition rises among the population. Childhood obesity is a particular risk as it often leads to adult obesity and chronic diseases later in life.

Dietitians need to continue to demonstrate the value they bring to helping solve the economic burden of rising health costs that are estimated to be in the billions each year. Recent estimates of the healthcare costs related to obesity alone are over $190 billion per year, or approximately 21 percent of all healthcare expenditures, and this does not include the cost of lost productivity, poor quality of life, or accommodations that must be made for equipment, seating, etc.[3]

PUBLIC HEALTH/COMMUNITY PRACTICE

Dietitians in community and public health areas work in many settings that focus on improving the health of population groups. Positions are characterized by an emphasis on health and wellness and the application of nutritional science. The dietitians may work in federal, state, or local public health agencies; neighborhood community health centers; industry; ambulatory health clinics; home health agencies and specialized community projects; nonprofit and for-profit private and community health agencies/institutions; private practice and hospitals; and public and private schools.

The Public Health/Community Nutrition Dietetic Practice Group describes the following wide variety of roles and settings in which dietitians work:[4]

- Providing population-based services at the national, state, and local level.
- Providing direct care in the Special Supplemental Nutrition Program for Women, Infants, and Children (WIC), primary care clinics, and other community-based settings.
- Serving as consultants to Head Start programs, child care centers, schools, school-based health clinics, home health programs, nursing homes, and other health care programs.
- Teaching in colleges, universities, and Cooperative Extension Service.
- Conducting research in academic and public health/community settings.
- Engaging in program planning, development, implementation, and evaluation at the federal, state, and local levels.
- Providing leadership and training in food safety, emergency preparedness, food security, and sustainable food and water systems.

The position paper "The Role of Health Promotion and Chronic Disease Prevention" also describes a range of activities dietitians perform in these areas.[5]

PUBLIC HEALTH NUTRITION

Every state has a department of health within state government employing public health dietitians. Many states use dietitians in programs such a Native American health service, Health and Human Services or welfare, departments of education, school nutrition programs, and in Area Agencies for the Aging.

The public health dietitian (or nutritionist) is usually required to have, at a minimum, the master's degree. He/she may not always be a registered dietitian nutritionist (RDN).

The full range of responsibilities of the public health dietitian includes familiarity with the field of public health. All segments of the population, including the healthy and those who are vulnerable to or experiencing chronic disease, are targeted. Assessment of health needs, applying preventive measures, and intervening with treatments and rehabilitation are core functions. This broader approach is distinguished from the clinical approach which more often concentrates on one-on-one assessment and care. Health promotion and disease prevention through service and research are requirements of all public health personnel.

The public health nutritionist establishes linkages with related community nutrition programs, nutrition education, food assistance, social or welfare services, and care services to the elderly. The public health approach has the following characteristics:[6]

- Interventions that promote health and prevent communicable and chronic diseases by managing or controlling the community environment.
- The promotion of a healthy lifestyle as a shared value for all people.
- Directing money and energy to the problems that affect the lives of the largest number of people in the community.
- Targeting the underserved or unserved by virtue of income, age, ethnicity, heredity, or lifestyle that are vulnerable to disease, hunger, or malnutrition.

- Collaboration of the public, community leaders, legislators, policy makers, administrators, and health and human services professionals in assessing and responding to community needs and consumer demands.
- Monitoring the nutritional health of the people in the community to ensure that the public health system achieves its objectives and responds to needs.

COMMUNITY NUTRITION

About 11 percent of RDNs and 12 percent of DTRs indicate their work area is in community nutrition. The Special Supplemental Nutrition Program for WIC employs 6 percent of the RDNs and 9 percent of the DTRs.[7] According to a 2012 membership survey of the PHCN DPG, some 45 percent of the respondents said community nutrition was their primary area of practice.[8]

Nutrition professionals in community nutrition usually acquire a general base of knowledge and a level of expertise in a chosen area (such as the needs of infants and children, pregnant women, older persons, or migrant individuals). The ability to use scientific methods to study, interpret, promote, and apply finding to community health problems through a knowledge of research is essential to practice. The community dietitian needs to understand the nutritional needs across the life cycle, use computer technology efficiently, and be aware of multiethnic needs and a diverse population. To be a credible nutrition resource, the RDN must understand the fundamentals of nutrition, food science, and dietetics, and have an underlying knowledge of human physiology, chemistry, biochemistry, epidemiology, statistics, and behavioral sciences. The RDN must also collaborate with community leaders and other professionals (such as social workers, public health nurses, rehabilitation specialists, pharmacists, teachers, store owners, etc.). Changing behavior by providing information about foods that are affordable and available in local market is a vital part of the counseling process.

Typical activities of the community nutrition RDN include the following:

- Assessment and prioritizing nutrition problems for various age and population groups.
- Ethical considerations in all programs and services offered.

- The integration of nutrition services into the overall agency mission, goals, and plans.
- Multidisciplinary and interdisciplinary team membership.
- Selection and/or development of nutrition education materials or approaches appropriate for individuals or small groups within the target population.
- Media strategies used in print, broadcasting, and telecommunications to reach population groups.
- Training of other agency staff and providing technical assistance to other staff.
- Serving as a resource to the public, media, business, and industry.

As noted earlier, over half the dietitians employed in community nutrition work in the WIC program. This program provides nutrition screening and nutrition education as well as food vouchers for low-income pregnant, breastfeeding and nonbreastfeeding women, and their children up to 5 years of age. The program is administered by the U.S. Department of Agriculture, which provides funding to state agencies for the program.

Other positions are in maternal and child nutrition, adult health, food service management, children with special needs and programs, day care programs for all ages, school nutrition, and programs in aging. Others may work in corrections institutions and in home care.

Another important area of practice in the community is in cooperative extension. This program is administered through land-grant colleges and universities in each state.[9] Personnel are employed at the county, district, and state levels. The primary responsibilities in this area of practice include planning, developing, and implementing nutrition, food, and health-related programs for all ages—4-H groups for young people as well as adult groups. Specialists in subject matter areas plan programs, provide specialized information, and help direct activities of county and district personnel.

In most states, the RDN credential may not be required for positions in cooperative extension. It is therefore a very promising area of practice for those who have not completed an internship or achieved the RD status.

CAREER OUTLOOK

Widespread concerns exist today within the public regarding the association of food and nutrition with other community/public health problems. The obesity epidemic and its complications continue to be a huge multifaceted problem with economic, medical, social, and psychological implications. Food availability, food safety, health disparities among ethnic groups, nutrition information, and misinformation are all impacting public health. The public health/community dietitian has an important role to play in helping meet these concerns. Involvement in policy decisions, obtaining advanced clinical skills, and advanced study in epidemiology and research methodology along with the use of evidence-based research are examples of ways the dietitian can help meet critical community health needs. In addition, networking and collaborating with other public health professionals is critical to success.[10,11] Dietitians who are prepared with managerial and conceptual skills as well as informatics will be increasingly needed in long-range program planning and policy implementation in communities.

The 2012 Member Survey by the PHCN DPG indicated a need for additional knowledge and skills acknowledged by the members who responded.[12] The following are areas indicated by 25 percent or more of the respondents:

- Community assessment
- Policy development
- Infant/child health
- Weight management
- Survey/surveillance and data

The list shows the forward thinking of the dietetic professionals currently working in community and public health nutrition.

SUMMARY

Public health/community nutrition encompasses a wide variety of programs and activities that impacts every segment of the population. Both food and feeding programs along with overall health maintenance and measures to prevent chronic diseases are the focus of professionals that work in these areas. State and federal programs target population groups who are underserved or unserved and dietitian/nutritionists provide nutrition surveillance, good feeding, and nutrition intake guidance, and collaborate with other professionals to provide service in these programs. Many opportunities are open for nutrition professionals in these areas of practice.

DEFINITIONS

Community health. Health measures applied to groups of people.
Community nutrition. Nutrition issues and services provided for groups of people.
Program planning. Needs assessment and action plans to meet needs.
Surveillance. Research-based activities to assess a program's reach and impact.

REFERENCES

1. American Dietetic Association. "Position of the American Dietetic Association: The Roles of Registered Dietitians and Diet Technicians in Health Promotion and Disease Prevention." *J Acad Nutr Diet* 113 (2013): 972–979.
2. Ibid.
3. Kaufman, M. *Nutrition in Promoting the Public Health: Strategies, Principles, and Practice.* (Sudbury, MA: Jones and Bartlett, 2007).
4. Public Health/Community Nutrition DPG. www.eatrightpro.org (2/25/16).
5. Slawson, D.L., N. Fitzgerald, and K.T. Morgan. "Position of the Academy of Nutrition and Dietetics: The Role of Nutrition in Health Promotion and Disease Prevention." *J Acad Nutr Diet* 113, no. 7 (2013): 972–979.
6. See Note 1.
7. Rogers, D. "Compensation and Benefits Survey 2015." *J Acad Nutr Diet* 116, no. 3 (2016): 370–388.
8. Public Health/Community Nutrition Practice Group 2012 Membership Survey Results. www.eatrightpro.org (3/15/16).
9. Chapman-Novakofski, K., and M. Reicks. "Dietetics Practitioners in Extension: What Is the Current Climate and Future Demand?" *J Acad Nutr Diet* 113, no. 10 (2013): 1875–1884.
10. Institute of Medicine. *Building Health Workforce Capacity through Community-Base Health Professional Education.* Workshop Summary. (Washington, DC: The National Academies Press, October 3, 2014).
11. See Note 10.
12. See Note 8.

CHAPTER 9

Dietitians in the Government and Military Services

"If dietetics is your profession, politics is your business."[1]

LEARNING OBJECTIVES

The student will be able to:

1. Name the largest federal government agencies related to food and nutrition.
2. Explain the differences and similarities between the Dietary Guidelines and Healthy People 2020.
3. Discuss ways the U.S. Department of Agriculture (USDA) provides food assistance to low-income groups.
4. Understand roles dietitians and dietetic technicians hold in government positions.
5. Describe how the dietary reference intakes (DRIs) are used and for what purposes.

PART I. THE GOVERNMENT

INTRODUCTION

Dietitians and nutritionists are employed in government activities and programs at the federal, state, and city or local levels. In 2015, about 6 percent of registered dietitian nutritionists (RDNs) and dietetic technicians, registered (DTRs) worked in government agencies and programs.[2] Even though the total number employed is small, all dietitians have vital interests in government activities because of the impact on professional practice in many areas of food, nutrition, and health, and many are actively involved in public policy through state legislative initiatives and support of national priorities.

Dietitians play a leading role in reaching the public about food, nutrition, and nutrition-related issues that are initiated by government agencies and/or by legislators. In doing so, the dietitian relies on his or her base of knowledge as well as on new and continuing information coming from research, food industry, and from the government. Congress passes legislation and government agencies issue guides and regulations that add to the bases of dietetic practice. For example, the Food and Nutrition Board of the National Research Council develops DRIs for the public, the Food and Drug Administration develops food labeling and food safety regulations, and the U.S. Department of Agriculture (USDA) and the Department of Health and Human Services (DHHS) issue food guides such as the Dietary Guidelines and MyPlate. These regulations and guides are important adjuncts to dietetic practice and nutrition education.

GOVERNMENT PROGRAMS IN FOOD AND NUTRITION

The USDA and DHHS are the two largest agencies of the government with the responsibility for the adequacy and safety of the food supply and for the health of all citizens. These objectives are realized through nutrition research, nutrition education, and food-related programs. The USDA has traditionally had the responsibility for food production, food consumption, and normal nutrition while the DHHS deals with the metabolic effects of dietary consumption patterns, particularly in relation to chronic disease.[3] There is overlap in these functions, but the agencies collaborate as well as conduct their specific programs and both are concerned with the nutritional health of all citizens.

The number of programs funded and administered by the government is extensive, and they deal with a broad range of activities concerned with the food supply, nutrition surveillance and monitoring, and recommendations for the public based on food surveys and research. The major programs in food and nutrition may be categorized as follows:

1. *National food and nutrition surveys.* The USDA has collected data on food intakes of individuals and families for many years. The "Continuing Survey of Food Intakes of Individuals" (CSFII) was a nationwide dietary survey beginning in 1985. The survey became part of the National Nutrition Monitoring System in 1990. In addition, the Diet and Health Knowledge Survey (DHKS) began in 1989 as a telephone survey using a personal interview questionnaire. Both these surveys were merged with the National Food and Nutrition Survey (NFNS) in 2002.

   The National Nutrition Monitoring and Related Research Act (NNMRR) was enacted by Congress in 1990 and is now conducted regularly. The law was passed to provide more organization and unification to existing survey methods and to coordinate the efforts of the 22 federal agencies that implement or review nutrition services and surveys.

Another national survey is conducted by the Centers for Disease Control and Prevention (CDC) called the National Health and Nutrition Examination Survey (NHANES). In this survey, about 6000 individuals are interviewed each year on food intakes followed by medical histories, physical measurements, and biochemical evaluations. Reports of the findings ae released each 2 years.

2. *Nutrition research.* Both the USDA and DHHS conduct research regarding nutrient content of foods, nutrient intakes, and the role of nutrition in treatment and prevention of disease. The National Institutes of Health (NIH), through research units within DHHS, conducts research in the major diseases and issue guidelines for dietary and nutritional management of many of the conditions.

The USDA sponsors research through grants to land-grant colleges and universities through the Agricultural Research Service. The department also conducts research at six centers around the country, an associated laboratory, and a research program in the Mississippi Delta. The research is focused on foods and the agricultural system and the effects on health, quality of life, and the promotion of a nutritious food supply.

The DHHS sponsors research through the NIH, a complex of 27 institutes and centers in Washington, DC, and on campuses throughout the country through intramural grants and programs. The NIH is described as the nation's medical research agency and represents the largest funded research source in the world. The focus of the research is to improve health and prevent disease. Many dietitian/nutritionists are employed in this agency.

3. *Food assistance and nutrition programs.* The National School Lunch and Breakfast Program, conducted by the USDA, provides free or reduced price meals in public, nonprofit private, and residential institutions. The national program is administered at the local level through state education agencies. Guidelines for foods served, based on the Dietary Guidelines, are developed by the Food and Nutrition Service. After-school snacks and summer feeding programs are also provided. Many dietitians are employed in school foodservice.

The Supplemental Nutrition Assistance Program (SNAP) is also conducted by the USDA. Funding by monthly food vouchers is provided to low-income households to purchase food from grocery stores or other sources such as farmer markets. Nutrition education is not a required part of this program although it is often provided to the clients by cooperative extension agents and community dietitians and nutritionists.

A large segment of community-based dietitians and nutritionists are employed in the Women's, Infants and Children's Program (WIC). Based usually in state or county health departments, the program provides foods as well as nutrition counseling and nutrition assessment to women during pregnancy and to children up to 5 years of age.

The nutrition program for the elderly provides a nutritious meal for older adults in congregate dining centers or through home-delivered meals. There is no income requirement for persons in this program and the programs are important for offering social contact as well as food for seniors.

4. *Food legislation and regulations.* The Food and Drug Administration issues guides for food safety, food labeling, and food additives, and monitors food in general. A grading system and labeling for meats and meat products is conducted by the USDA. The CDC monitors and collects data on food-related illnesses and issues recommendations for the public. Several other agencies such as the Environmental Protection Agency and the Federal Trade Commission that also monitor food advertising issue regulations regarding food and food safety. All these departments function to develop their regulations based on legislation enacted by Congress.

5. *Dietary guidelines for the public.* The two large agencies—USDA and DHHS—appoint a scientific committee each 5 years to review the evidence and make recommendations for current Dietary Guidelines for Americans. The guidelines focus on good eating practices in terms of best food choices and foods and nutrient to be avoided or reduced. The latter are primarily sodium, fat, and sugar while those recommended are ones containing fiber, complex carbohydrates, and plant-based proteins. Exercise and safe food handling and, in 2015, an emphasis on the whole diet pattern are all part of the guidance. The two agencies issue the final

recommendations that are incorporated into the school foodservice program, community nutrition programs, and many others. "Healthy People" is published at 10-year intervals by the DHHS focusing on total health of the U.S. population. Currently working toward the 2020 goals of the program, the targets are nutrition and weight, heart disease and stroke, diabetes, oral health, cancer, and healthy aging. Specific objectives are developed, which are evaluated at the midpoint of each decade to assess progress toward the goals.

Recommended dietary allowances (RDAs) were first developed in 1943 and were updated at approximate 10-year intervals thereafter. In 1998, the pattern changed with the issuance of a group of guidelines known as *dietary reference intakes* (DRIs) that are now the standards for nutrient intakes for individuals and groups by age, sex, and activity. The guides are developed by the Food and Nutrition Board of the National Research Council.

6. *Nutrition education.* Nutrition education for the public is extensive and varied. The translation of dietary guidance into specific eating patterns is the responsibility of the Center for Nutrition Policy and Promotion in the USDA. The current pattern is the MyPlate, a pictorial representation of the recommended eating plan. Guides for using the plan are also issued. There have been other plans in the past such as the Food Pyramid and Basic Four and Basic Seven. Other information sources provided by the USDA are the National Nutrient Databank, the National Evidence Library, and the National Agriculture Library that supplies information worldwide. DHHS maintains the National Medical Library with the NIH to provide disease prevention and treatment information to the public as well as to researchers and professionals in the medical and allied health fields.

At the state level, dietitians in public health nutrition are employees of state health departments and conduct nutrition and health education programs in the community. Dietitians in the Indian Health Service work in state programs administered by the Federal Office of Indian Affairs. Nutrition education for individuals and families is also conducted through the cooperative extension service at land-grant colleges and universities.

Agencies administering school food service programs, the food stamp program, and the elderly nutrition programs vary from state to state. However, the programs are all similar and meet the same national standards. The national network of federal, state, and local cooperative extension personnel "extend" research and pertinent information from the government and the educational institutions to the public.

ROLE OF THE ACADEMY OF NUTRITION AND DIETETICS IN POLICY FORMATION

Washington Office

The Academy became active in governmental and legislative affairs in the 1960s and now has a very effective network in place. A Washington office is staffed in part with persons who are registered as lobbyists on behalf of the Association. The staff monitors legislative developments in food and nutrition and practice-related issues and works closely with the Department of Government and Legal Affairs in the Chicago headquarters office to promote the association's priorities for action. A volunteer legislative and public policy team, appointed by the Board of Directors, works with both offices to gain information from states and members and, in turn, transmit information back to states and members about pending public policy actions.

Public Policy Workshop

A workshop is conducted by the Washington and Chicago headquarters staff each year to inform members of pending legislation, to help them become knowledgeable about the political process and to make contacts with legislators and other government officials. Currently, the workshop is offered by live streaming television, affording two-way interaction with members.

Position and Practice Papers

Another important way the Association provides policy input is through position and practice papers developed by members and approved for publication by the House of Delegates. The papers represent a *consensus of viewpoints and professional interests and are used in many ways such as media contacts*, in contacting legislators, and with the public. Papers are periodically updated or deleted if the information is out of date or no longer relevant.

Examples of current position and practice papers that are particularly pertinent to policy issues are the following[4]:

- Healthy Food Choices
- Nutrition and Disease Prevention: Intervention and Management
- Nutrition Through the Life Span
- Safeguarding the Public
- Nutrition and Women's Health
- Promoting Ecologic Sustainability within the Food System
- Using the DRIs

Position papers issued by the Academy may be accessed at www .eatright.org

Legislative Network Coordinators

Each state designates a legislative chair and a legislative network coordinator (LNC), who coordinate legislative activities among Academy members in the state. The LNC helps prepare other volunteers who use prepared talking points in contacts with members. In addition, grassroot liaisons (GRL) are designated in each state who are assigned to one or more legislators to work with them directly in advocating for Academy positions.

Political Action Committee

The Academy of Nutrition and Dietetics Political Action Committee (ANDPAC) receives voluntary contributions from members for the purpose of promoting legislative action on issues of concern. The monies received are used to make a yearly contribution to a Congressman or woman who has been instrumental in forwarding Association public policy concerns. The designee is recognized at the annual meeting of the Academy.

POLICY ISSUES IN DIETETICS

Public policy and advocacy are core functions of the Academy and crucial to achieving the mission, vision, goals, and strategies of the Association. Public policy influences the public image of the Academy and its members as well as the successful implementation of actions the Association stands for—better health for all citizens.

Academy groups and members work on a broad range of issues. For focus and guidance regarding policy issues, several priority areas are identified:[5]

- Disease prevention and treatment, including cancer, cardiovascular disease, diabetes and pre-diabetes, HIV/AIDS, obesity and weight, access to health care.
- Lifecycle nutrition, including prenatal and maternal health, early childhood nutrition, school-age students, and nutrition for older adults.
- Quality health care, including healthcare equity, consumer protection and licensure, workforce demand, research and monitoring, lowering healthcare costs, and quality measures.
- Medical nutrition therapy (MNT) has been a legislative priority in the Academy leading to its initial passage by Congress in the 1990s. By continuing to work closely with the Centers for Medicare and Medicaid Services (CMS), specific issues are addressed pertaining to the role of RDNs in the management of illness or injury. Reimbursement for services provided by the dietitian/nutritionist is an objective.[6]

PART II. THE MILITARY SERVICES

Military service is another area of practice for dietitians in the government. Dietitians are employed in the army, navy, and air force where they function in very similar activities as in many other areas of dietetics. Most work in hospitals throughout the United States and in other countries and have positions in clinical dietetics, food service management, and community nutrition. Others are in research, in personnel recruiting, and in health promotion.

Dietitians in the military service meet the education and experience requirements of the Academy and are registered. They receive basic military training, as in a field hospital, for readiness in the event of war or military action. They are commissioned officers and can expect to progress in rank and salary as well as in positions over time.

In the army, dietetic interns and dietitians are members of the Army Medical Specialist Corps. In the air force, they are members of the U.S. Air Force Biomedical Science Corps. In the navy, most work in hospitals in the United States and elsewhere where military personnel are stationed.

At the entry level, duties of the dietitian include providing nutrition assessments and counseling for inpatients, consultation with child care and schools located on military bases, and nutrition/health promotion for the military community. Other job duties may include supervising food production and service. The entry-level dietitian is often responsible for personnel management of a small military staff and civilian staff depending on the position. Senior dietitians are more often involved in establishing policy that affects the nutritional health of soldiers and their families.

A U.S. Military Dietetic Internship Consortium is offered in Texas, which combines a master's degree with the internship. Course work for the degree is offered at Baylor University and supervised practice may be taken at one of three locations: Fort Sam Houston, San Antonio Medical Center, Walter Reed National Military Center in Bethesda, or the Madigan Army Medical Center at Fort Lewis, Washington. The master's degree is awarded by Baylor University.

Army dietitians, as commissioned officers, are paid and promoted based on their military rank. Housing and food allowances are also provided based on geographic location. Promotions are dependent on education (advanced degrees), military education (the Army offers officer/leader development courses), and job performance. An advantage of the military promotion system is that a dietitian may change job position or location without a loss of seniority. Military dietitians can expect to relocate at intervals, and with each move, there are opportunities for varied positions. Continuing education to maintain RD eligibility as well as for continued self-development is highly encouraged.

A history of military dietitians in the Association and their service was published in the *Journal of the Academy* in 2014.[7]

SUMMARY

Dietitians are employed in the government at national, state, and local levels. They are involved in legislation and develop position and practice papers as well as contributing to a PAC. They participate in food and nutrition research and provide nutrition education for the public. They are commissioned officers in the military services providing nutritional care and food services for military personnel and families.

Activities of the Academy on behalf of dietitians include promotion of policy issues important to the profession and education of dietitians in legislative activities. Dietitians are involved in policy making through contacts with legislators and in support of Association activities that further the profession of dietetics and benefit the public.

DEFINITIONS

Food Assistance. Food that is provided in feeding programs or by voucher to buy food.

Political Action Committee. Group pooling of money to support political candidates or office holders.

Public Policy. The promotion of a law, a regulation, or a recommendation targeted to the public at large.

Regulation. Written rules to activate laws passed through legislation.

REFERENCES

1. Washington Report. ADA Courier. 35, no. 9 (1996): 1.
2. Rogers, D. "Compensation and Benefits Survey 2015." *J Acad Nutr Diet* 116, no. 3 (2016): 370–388.
3. www.eatright.org/advocacy (11/23/15).
4. The Academy of Nutrition and Dietetics. "Position and Practice Paper Update." *J Acad Nutr Diet* 115, no. 2 (2015): 284–285.
5. Eatright.org (11/23/15).
6. Neidert, K. "Advocating at the Centers for Medicare and Medicaid Services." *J Acad Nutr Diet* 113, no. 4 (2013): 505–507.
7. Stein, K. "The Academy's Military Roots Visualized." *J Acad Nutr Diet* 114, no. 12 (2014): 2023–2049.

CHAPTER 10

The Consultant in Health Care, Business, and Private Practice

"Entrepreneurs shape the future dietetics practice by pursuing innovative and creative ways of providing nutrition products and services."[1]

OUTLINE

· Ethical and Legal Bases of Practice
· Summary
· Definitions
· References

LEARNING OBJECTIVES

The student will be able to:

1. Become familiar with personal characteristics needed to become a consultant.
2. Develop a resume if not already completed.
3. Gain knowledge about setting fees, negotiating contracts, and obtaining liability insurance.
4. Become familiar with federal, state, and local regulations pertaining to consulting in healthcare facilities.
5. Understand in general the responsibilities of the consultant in health care.
6. Understand consultation in business and the variety of options available.
7. Become familiar with the range of opportunities available in private practice.

INTRODUCTION

As a result of the 2015 Compensation and Benefits Survey, it was reported that 8 percent of registered dietitians (RDs) and about 2 percent of dietetic technicians, registered (DTRs) indicated their primary practice area was in consultation and business.[2] Many dietitians have found the schedule flexibility and compensation of self-employment attractive alternatives to more traditional positions. An entrepreneurial drive is often the impetus for a professional to become a consultant and/or establish a practice. Others do so because family or other obligations lead to becoming a consultant for a better lifestyle fit.

Healthcare institutions have moved an increasing number of services from inpatient care into outpatient clinics, other community agencies, or home care. Governmental regulations led to the need for nutrition consultants in extended care facilities in the 1970s. Together, these trends have led to the need for a greater number of consultant dietitians.

Three types of consultant practice are discussed in this chapter, and while there are similar characteristics of the successful practitioner as in many of the job requirements, each area is unique in several ways because of the nature of the business or practice. The practice areas are consultants in health care and extended care, such as nursing homes and long-term care institutions, consultants in business, and consultants in private practice.

BECOMING A CONSULTANT

Starting a practice as a consultant requires forethought and planning. Two very helpful publications available to guide the dietitian in planning are Helm's *The Entrepreneurial Dietitian* and *The Competitive Edge*.[3,4]

The first step is self-assessment. Personal characteristics are important because an entrepreneur needs to be self-directed, energetic, and action oriented. Previous working experience in dietetics is very important for the person considering becoming a consultant because a great deal of independent activity and judgment is needed, and success is dependent on having had opportunities to develop these characteristics. A number of questions leading to an assessment of a person's readiness for practice are the following:[5]

- Are you a self-starter?
- Are you a risk taker?
- Do you have a positive, friendly interest in others?
- Are you a leader?
- Can you handle responsibility?
- Are you a good organizer?
- Are you able to handle a flexible working schedule?
- Do you make up your mind quickly?
- Can people rely on you?
- Can you handle reversals and downturns in business?

A professional making a career change to consulting may need to update his or her resume. It is important to tailor the resume in a way that emphasizes experience and professional qualifications, highlighting those skills that pertain most closely to the position being planned. The resume should be concise, should use strong action verbs, and should be specific about past experiences. Examples of resumes for several different career areas are shown by Matthieu.[6]

Employers look for workers with skills as well as knowledge and specific competencies. A comprehensive discussion of competency-based hiring gives helpful guides to the job expectations and interview.[7]

The interview will be a next important step after the resume has been sent and after one or more call-backs from interested clients. A professional attitude and appearance make a good first impression. Some advance research about the company or facility will help to formulate additional questions and show interest. Discussion of the amount of time, contracts, and pay should come in the later part of the interview.[8]

Networking with other successful dietitians through one or more practice groups is an excellent way of gaining valuable start-up information. Mentors may be found and networks established from these contacts. Professional liability insurance should be considered early in the planning stage. This insurance is available through the office of the Academy of Nutrition and Dietetics. Networking is also a way of obtaining accounts or positions. Initiating contacts with a healthcare facility or business is followed by a meeting with the administrator and other key personnel. Negotiations should include a clear understanding of the amount of time the consultant will be needed. Although regulations in a healthcare institution may require a dietetic consultant only a small number of hours per month, there may be compelling reasons for more time to be spent in the facility. For instance, in institutions with a large number of residents or in institutions in which a number of residents require skilled care, additional consultation time may well be needed.

Contracts and Fees

Major considerations for the dietitian in consultation and private practice are setting prices and fees and obtaining reimbursement for services. These will be spelled out in the contract, which is a legal document outlining the obligations between the parties involved.[9] Establishing and negotiating the ground rules are important in the initial stages of the process.

Consultants can gain information about reimbursement rates by researching pay levels in the area and region for different types of consulting work and for basic salary levels. Networking with others in a practice group is a good way of obtaining information regarding typical fees. Dietitians who receive reimbursement from insurers or hospitals for medical nutrition therapy (MNT) will be guided by MNT codes establishing payment for treatments authorized by Medicare.[10]

Expenses such as liability insurance, mileage, travel, and any educational components needed should be added to the base pay to arrive at a fee.[11] Ethical billing practices are pointed out in an article by Horowitz and White.[11]

THE CONSULTANT IN HEALTH CARE AND EXTENDED CARE

The role of the consultant in healthcare facilities and extended care became important with the enactment of the Medicare regulations by the Centers for Medicare and Medicaid Services or (CMS). The Omnibus Reconciliation Act of 1987, amended in 1990 and 1993, provided regulations for nutritional care in long-term facilities that received federal Medicare funds.[12] These facilities (primarily nursing homes) were required to hire a qualified dietitian; as a result, the demand for consultant dietitians rapidly increased from a limited employment area with a short history, few guidelines, and dietitians on their own insofar as job requirements and benefits were concerned. Consultation in healthcare facilities became areas in which many dietitians soon found employment. The opportunities helped many dietitians who had been out of the workforce to return to practice. Some of these dietitians needed to be updated in practice knowledge and skills and turned to continuing education opportunities to refresh themselves on necessary information to practice. Today, many dietitians work as consultants in nursing homes and small hospitals funded by federal and state agencies.

Federal regulations state that the consultant's visits should be of "sufficient frequency to meet the food and nutrition needs of residents in the facility."[13] In many facilities, this meant a minimum of 8 hours a month. While the federal regulations were vague in regard to the actual amount of time required, many states, through licensing, require a minimum of 8 hours. A dietitian contracts with a facility for the amount of time needed, at or above the minimum, to meet the facility's needs.

Some consultants contract with more than one facility and may thereby work part time or full time as they choose. Some dietitians are employed full time for a multifacility chain or in one large facility.

Regulations

A consultant must be familiar with state and federal regulations that apply to long-term or extended care facilities. The health department in each state can provide copies of both regulations. Federal regulations are precise concerning both the physical plant and operations as well as staffing. Each facility has its own procedures and set of regulations governing operations. The consultant needs to be thoroughly familiar with these as well as the policies and goals of the facility.

All healthcare providers in the United States need to be familiar with the Health Insurance Portability and Accountability Act (HIPAA) of 1996, as this set of rules concerning rights of patients and clients must be addressed and clients notified of the facility's privacy procedures.[14]

Areas of Practice

Long-term facilities include nursing homes, skilled nursing facilities, subacute care centers, adult day care, residential care facilities, and alcohol and drug rehabilitation facilities. Long-term care facilities may be owned privately, by the cities or counties, by religious organizations, or by corporations. They may be for profit or not for profit; the number of beds varies.

Consultants also may be hired to visit developmentally disabled clients in their homes. In addition, some state health departments contract with consultants to provide services for Women, Infants, and Children (WIC) participants. Other consultants work in home health care, congregate feeding sites, senior citizen centers, correctional facilities, group homes for the developmentally disabled, hospice programs, and small rural hospitals. Adult day care, group homes, and retirement communities are other facilities offering opportunities for the consultant dietitian in health care.

Roles and Responsibilities

A consultant functions in an advisory capacity within a facility; however, he or she has ethical and professional responsibilities for the nutritional care of the residents. Ethical practice issues must be guided by the Academy's code of ethics. Professional responsibilities are delineated in the *ADA Standards of Practice for Professional Performance for Registered Dietitians in Nutrition Care*[15] and the *ADA Standards of Practice of Practice and Standards of Professional Performance for Registered Dietitians (Competent, Proficient, and Expert) in Extended Care Settings.*[16] By developing rapport and using organizational skills, the consultant is able to accomplish the needed tasks. Because he or she is usually not in the facility full time, the day-to-day supervision of dietary services may be provided by a DTR or a dietetic manager.

When a consultant begins employment in a facility, one of the first activities should be to need to assess of the food and nutrition services for the residents. This assessment will guide further planning and action. Documentation of observations and plans for future visits are very important, beginning with the first visit. The typical activities a consultant performs during a visit to a facility include the following:

- Conferring with the dietary manager and the administrator about day-to-day operations and any problems that need to be addressed during the visit
- Performing nutrition assessment of new residents and conducting a follow-up for all others
- Checking at-risk residents and making recommendations for further nutritional care as indicated. This includes noting unexplained changes in weight or the development of pressure ulcers, checking those on tube feedings, and noting signs of dehydration or otherwise poor nutritional status
- Observing the meal service and eating a meal to evaluate food quality
- Making nutrition rounds and visiting the group dining area at meal time to observe the residents' acceptance of the food and their food intake
- Conducting educational in-service sessions for employees and exchange information regarding departmental activities
- Documenting all activities with any recommendations for follow-up

The consultant may be responsible for developing policy and procedure manuals for the quality improvement program, for safety and sanitation procedures, and for budget management. The reference diet manual should be reviewed and signed by the chief of the medical staff at least annually and should be updated regularly. Consultants may also teach dietetic technician students, conduct classes for the dietary manager, and serve as a preceptor for students in supervised experiences in long-term care.

Standards for Quality Assurance

The dietetics in health care communities dietetic practice group developed standards of practice in 2011 as a guide for quality assurance in practice.[17] The standards specify areas of activity with examples of outcomes. They include the provision of services, application of research, communication and application of knowledge, utilization and management of resources, and continued competence and professional accountability.

Through written documentation, consultant dietitians can verify actual performance and implement action to meet the expected outcomes. The standards also help develop a workable plan to help consultants meet the responsibilities for which they have been contracted and to evaluate their own knowledge, clinical experience, and management expertise.

THE CONSULTANT IN BUSINESS PRACTICE

An increasingly popular area of practice for the dietitian with an entrepreneurial drive is in business and nontraditional career areas. Potential practice areas identified by the Nutrition Entrepreneurs practice group include services for individuals, corporations, the media, restaurants, food companies, Internet and business technology, sports and health facilities, and coaching. Other areas are in pharmaceutical sales, medical and institutional equipment sales, catering, chefs' schools, and specialized clinics.

Dietitians who work as consultants in businesses of all kinds like to take on new challenges and are often described as risk takers in new areas of practice. They are energetic and versatile individuals with backgrounds and experience preparing them for innovative roles—roles they may even be required to create. Although many of the responsibilities of a consultant may be similar to those for a full-time dietitian, one of the main differences is often the duration of the assignment. In an established business, the consultant may be given a short-term contract with an identified scope of work and specific deliverables (outcomes). The scope of services is usually an assignment to set up or improve the business practices of the client. It also may be a specific project with a defined beginning and end time period. Examples of activities the consultant may perform include evaluating staffing patterns, establishing an inventory and cost-control system, planning a new production or service system, recommending equipment purchases, and establishing a computerized control system.

Areas of Practice

Business consulting firms at times employ entry-level dietitians for consulting, usually within a defined scope of responsibility. More often, the dietitian is experienced in some area (e.g., as a clinical dietitian in a healthcare facility or manager of a food service system). The dietitian may have also worked as an assistant with other dietitian for a food processor equipment manufacturer, publisher, marketing company, or software company. When hired, he or she may first be assigned to a team leader to work on a specific part of a major project. With experience, there may be opportunities to expand into other nontraditional roles such as facility management, accounting, design, sales, or marketing. The range of responsibility is dependent on the scope of the services performed by the company and those that the dietitians can develop for the company.

The following guidelines can be used by those who may be considering moving into management with the goal of consultation in business, private practice, or health care:

- Consider one's personal qualifications for independent action
- Seek advice from a veteran manager or other mentors
- Join a practice group for networking and sharing
- Become familiar with the mission and goals of the business or health-care organization
- Keep up-to-date with the professional literature and continuing education opportunities
- Take advantage of the evidence-based library resources
- Consider further education if advancement and pay would benefit
- Attend professional seminars and meetings
- Be familiar with and apply all aspects of ethical practice
- Match job requirements with education and experience
- Be proficient in the use of technology
- Seek ways to constantly evaluate personal performance

Communications through use of social media is increasingly important in consultations of all kinds, including business. Ethical considerations must be a part of this usage as outlined in an ethics opinion by the Academy.[18]

THE CONSULTANT IN PRIVATE PRACTICE

Many dietitians today become entrepreneurs and enter private practice for a variety of reasons. Some seek new and innovative opportunities out of choice; others do so due to circumstances that make private practice an attractive choice. Examples of the latter might be the loss of a job or the need to work varying hours because of family responsibilities. Opportunities for women in the business world are unquestionably increasing. The healthcare industry continues to downsize from large, centralized centers to outpatient and community centers with fewer staff. Many dietitians seek greater independence and new challenges and, along with a business climate that encourages entrepreneurs, find satisfying careers in private practice.

Not all consultants start a business. Some work at home and combine home and family responsibilities with part-time, contract-type work such as writing, preparing marketing and educational materials, computer searches, and home visits. If a decision is made to open an office, appropriate equipment must be obtained, and secretarial help, as well as other assistants or an office manager, will need to be considered.

Starting a Practice

Cross[19] provides a helpful checklist for starting a private practice. The first step, she points out, is to maintain an updated file of one's professional credentials and achievements. Regarding references, both giving and receiving employment references may present important issues to be considered.[20] Obtaining state licensure or certification and keeping professional credentials up to date helps establish qualifications. Joining the state association, dietetic practice groups, and specialty groups, if applicable, will provide opportunities for networking. Becoming involved in local business groups or taking business classes helps one learn the business climate.

Creating a vision and finding one's focus, then creating the road map or business plan, is the next step.[21] The business plan should incorporate the mission and vision statement, product or service to be provided, a description of the target market, the competition, and financial projections. Identifying where to find professional support from an accountant, a banker, a marketing specialist, an information technology specialist, and perhaps a lawyer will provide valuable assistance. Banks, investment companies, and community small-business start-up programs often provide advice to assist entrepreneurs in starting a business.

Establishing the business basics by estimating expenses, obtaining necessary insurance, and writing policies and procedures are important steps. A marketing program and a quality-assurance program will help launch and maintain the business. The benefits that can be realized from careful planning include seeing clients succeed and realizing a business profit.

The dietitian who enters private practice needs to possess confidence, determination, perseverance, and the motivation to remain current on trends and changes in the profession and the business world. Remaining up to date comes in great part through taking advantage of continuing education opportunities. The Nutrition Entrepreneurs practice group advises anyone going into private practice—whether to write a book, start a business, become a speaker or coach, or use the Internet to market or provide products and services—to find help through a mentor, and it offers participation in a mentorship program.

Areas of Practice

The consultant in private practice usually will be located outside an organization, but also may be an intrapreneur, or one within an organization who develops new ideas or services that are used profitably in some way. The potential work settings are as diverse as the practitioner's interests and expertise as well as the market demand. This variety is illustrated in **Table 10-1**.

The professional services provided are influenced by the needs of the consumer, the demands and changing environments of health care, changes in regulatory agencies, increased autonomy, and advances in science and technology.[22] As new ideas are disseminated and needs identified, more roles are defined for the private practitioner. Dietitians may form alliances and networks to provide services. By teaming with other professionals, the ability to market services and products and share business expense is enhanced. The opportunities presented through a wider range of contacts also may be increased. Examples of such associations are dietitian networks and dietitian-independent practice associations. Dietetic practice groups provide a means for networking among professionals.

Practice Roles

Consultants in private practice may teach clients and consumers in areas ranging from wellness and prevention to MNT, business and industry,

Table 10-1.   Settings for Consulting in Private Practice

Private office

Media and communications

Private home

Grocery stores

Physician's or other allied health professional's office

Restaurants and culinary industry

Corporate settings of work sites

Home health care

Business and industry

Health/fitness/wellness centers and spas

Food companies

Community-based programs

Hotels and resorts

Schools

Research centers

Hospitals

Medical education consulting firms

Day and group homes

Private specialty clinic (specializing in sports medicine, eating disorders, diabetes, renal diseases, oncology, HIV/AIDS)

Senior citizen centers

Nursing homes

Governmental contracts

Rehabilitation centers

Child development centers

Assisted living facilities

Retirement centers

Adapted from Alexander-Israel, D., and C. Roman-Shriver. In *Dietetics: Practice and Future Trends*, 3rd ed. E.A. Winterfeldt, M.L. Bogle, and L.L. Ebro. (Gaithersburg, MD: Aspen Publishers, 2011), p. 137.

food service and culinary trades, and writing and media presentation. A list of activities is shown in **Table 10-2** as examples of the types of services that consultants may perform.

Practice roles often can be expanded with more training in business, marketing, and communications and with the development of new skills that cross the boundaries into other health professions.[23] For example,

Table 10-2.   Roles of Consultants in Private Practice

Assessment of nutritional status

Menu evaluation and planning

Recipe evaluation and modification

One-on-one counseling

Family counseling

Group counseling

Monitoring of nutritional intervention

Dietary analysis and evaluation of products

Consultant to agencies, institutions, and programs with nutrition components, such as extended care, school food service, hospitals, government agencies, or clinics

Consultant to professionals (health care, food service, culinary industry)

Consultant to corporations (fitness centers, wellness/health promotion programs, benefits departments)

Writing for the lay public (books, newsletters, magazines, newspaper articles)

Professional publications

Group training, presentations, workshops

Developing nutritious/healthier menu items for restaurants

Restaurant and culinary staff training

Assistance in marketing nutrition in restaurants

Computer/software programming (quality management, nutrition education, food service, clinical nutrition)

Developing and marketing nutrition education programs (private and public)

Supermarket tours and grocery information guides

Nutrition labeling information

Rehabilitation and sports injury consultation

Nutrition care planning

Monitoring compliance with local, state, federal regulations (long-term care facilities, drug and alcohol centers, prisons)

Developing, administering, and evaluating nutrition standards

Multidisciplinary preventive and therapeutic services

Health coaching

Data from Alexander-Israel, D., and C. Roman-Shriver. In *Dietetics: Practice and Future Trends.* E.A. Winterfeldt, M.L. Bogle, and L.L. Ebro. (Gaithersburg, MD: Aspen Publishers, 1998), p. 209.

dietitians can become proficient at taking blood pressure and body composition measurements in the home care setting; can secure American College of Sports Medicine Exercise Test Technology certification for performing electrocardiogram-monitored stress tests in sports medicine clinics, or Clinical Laboratory Certification for blood analysis; or can use phlebotomy skills in wellness programs.

Continually emerging roles demand expansion of the dietitian's scope of practice and skills and capitalizing on the talents that are unique to dietitians. Among these are the ability to apply food and nutrition knowledge, use nutrition assessment tools, apply lifestyle-change education to prevent or manage disease, and to collect data on outcomes of nutrition intervention on quality of life and overall care costs.

ETHICAL AND LEGAL BASES OF PRACTICE

The *Code of Ethics for the Profession of Dietetics* is the primary document governing ethical practice in all areas of dietetics. This document, along with any applicable rules or statutes of practice, including licensure from state and local authorities, should be familiar to all consultants. These guidelines will clarify the responsibilities to the public, to clients, to the profession, and to colleagues and other professionals. Feeney[24] offers practical tips for the dietitian applying the code to ethical practice when questions or conflicts arise. Grandgenett[25] gives specific case examples of ethical dilemmas in business practice with discussion of ways they can be handled.

As discussed earlier, the consultant may need to retain legal advice at the outset in order to negotiate a contract and other job-related provisions. The contract is a legal document that guides the consultant's scope of practice and may serve as a template for later functions. All consultants should carry personal liability insurance to protect against the possibility of legal action arising out of job-related activities.

SUMMARY

Traditional institutional roles for dietitians, especially in clinical dietetics, are still predominant practice settings; however, many dietitians are using their clinical background to become entrepreneurs in their own practice. The dietitian who possesses the needed personal attributes and the initiative and creativity needed for entrepreneurial success may find a rewarding new career in consultation in healthcare facilities, businesses, or private practice.

DEFINITIONS

Client. The recipient of services or products.

Consultant. A skilled and knowledgeable person qualified to give expert professional advice.

Entrepreneur. An innovative person who initiates a new activity, career, or business.

Intrapraneur. A person within an organization who develops new ideas or services.

Long-term care. Assistance provided over time to people with chronic health conditions and/or physical disabilities and those who are unable to care for themselves.

Managed care. A system of care administered by an entity outside a hospital or healthcare institution in which access, cost, and quality of care are controlled by direct intervention before or during service for purposes of creating efficiencies and/or reducing costs.

Nutrition assessment. Evaluation of an individual's nutritional status based on anthropometric, biochemical, clinical, and dietary information.

Private practice. Self-employment in which a person manages his or her own working career.

Quality improvement. The provision of service that assures the needs of those served are met through adherence to high standards of care.

REFERENCES

1. Academy of Nutrition and Dietetics. *Nutrition Entrepreneurs Dietetic Practice Group.* (2012).

2. Rogers, D. "Compensation and Benefits Survey 2015." *J Acad Nutr Diet* 115, no. 3 (2015): 20.

3. Helm, K.K. *The Entrepreneurial Nutritionist*, 4th ed. (Lake Dallas, TX: K.K. Helm Publications, 2010).

4. Helm, K.K. *The Competitive Edge. Advanced Marketing for Dietetic Professionals*, 3rd ed. (Chicago: The Academy of Nutrition and Dietetics, 2009).

5. Adapted from: Cross, A.T. "Practical and Legal Considerations of Private Nutrition Practice." *J Am Diet Assoc* 95 (1995): 21–29.

6. Matthieu, J. "Revamping Your Resume for Your Specialty." *J Am Diet Assoc* 110 (2010): 353–355.

7. Peregrin, T. "Competency Based Hiring: The Key to Recruiting and Retaining Successful Employees." *J Acad Nutr Diet* 114, no. 9 (2014): 1330–1339.

8. McCafree, J. "Contract Basics: What a Dietitian Should Know." *J Acad Nutr Diet* 103 (2003): 429–440.

9. Peregrin, T. "From Contracts to Clean Claim: Guidelines for Getting Paid." *J Am Diet Assoc* 110 (2010): 837–839.

10. Bender, T. "2009 Medicare MNT Payment Information." *Ventures* XXV, no. 4 (2009): 10.

11. Hodorowicz, M.A., and J.V. White. "Elements of Ethical Billing for Nutritional Professionals." *J Acad Nutr Diet* 112, no. 3 (2012): 432–435.

12. Omnibus Budget Reconciliation Act 1987. Amended 1990, 1993.

13. "Skilled Nursing Facilities: Standards for Certification and Participation in Medicare and Medicaid Programs." *Federal Register* 39 (1974): 22–38.

14. Boyce, B. "HIPAA Compliance from a Private Practice Per View." *J Acad Nutr Diet* 114, no. (9), 2014: 1341–1346.

15. American Dietetic Association Quality Management Committee. "American Dietetic Association Revised 2008 Standards of Practice for Registered Dietitians in Nutrition; Standards of Professional Practice for Registered Dietitians; Standards of Practice for Dietetic Technicians, Registered, in Nutrition Care; and Standards of Professional Performance for Dietetic Technicians, Registered." *J Am Diet Assoc* 108 (2008): 1538–1542.

16. Roberts, L., S.C. Cryst, G.E. Robinson, C.H. Robinson, C.H. Elliott, L.C. Moore, M. Rybicki, and M.P. Carlson. "American Dietetic Association: Standards of Practice and Standards of Professional Performance for Registered Dietitians (Competent, Proficient, and Expert) in Extended Care Settings." *J Am Diet Assoc* 11 (2011): e617–624, e627.

17. See Note 16.

18. Ayres, E.J. "The Impact of Social Media on Business and Ethical Practices in Dietetics." *J Acad Nutr Diet* 113, no. (11): 1539–1543.

19. Cross, M. "Getting Started in Private Practice: A Checklist to Your Entrepreneurial Path." *J Am Diet Assoc* 108 (2008): 21–24.

20. Zackin, F.M. "Employment References—Giving and Receiving." *J Am Diet Assoc* 108 (2008): 1053–1055.

21. See Note 8.

22. ADA. "The Role of Dietetics Professional in Health Promotion and Disease Prevention." *J Am Diet Assoc* 102 (2002): 1680–1687.

23. See Note 6.

24. Feeney, M.J. "When Ethics Collide: An independent Dietetic Consultant's Perspective on Balancing Professional Ethics with the Wishes of Your Client." *J Am Diet Assoc* 108 (2008): 29–31.

25. Grandgenett, R. "Ethics in Business Practice." *J Am Diet Assoc* 110 (2010): 1103–1104.

CHAPTER 11

Career Choices in Business, Communications, and Health and Wellness

"The ancient Greeks attained a high level of civilization based on good nutrition, regular physical activity, and intellectual development."[1]

OUTLINE

- Learning Objectives
- Introduction
- The Dietitian in Business and Communications
  - Career Opportunities
  - Mentors and Networks
  - Strategic Skill Building
- The Dietitian in Health and Wellness Programs
  - Sports Nutrition
  - Cardiovascular Nutrition
  - Wellness and Health Promotion
  - Disordered Eating
- Practice Groups
- Summary
- Definitions
- References

LEARNING OBJECTIVES

The student will be able to:

1. Discuss the wide range of employment opportunities in business.
2. Describe areas of practice in health and wellness, sports, and specialty areas in medical nutrition.
3. Gain awareness of the communication skills needed by the successful consultant.
4. Gain appreciation for the personal characteristics helpful in the business world.
5. Understand the importance of networking and mentors in making employment decisions.

INTRODUCTION

Hospitals and extended care facilities have long been the work settings for the largest percentage of dietitians and dietetic technicians; however, other potential career choices are emerging in other settings. This movement is in part because of the creativity in education and the changing needs for nutrition information. Consultation and private practice were discussed in a previous chapter. In this chapter, three additional general areas of dietetic practice potential and opportunity are presented: business, communications, and health and wellness.

THE DIETITIAN IN BUSINESS AND COMMUNICATIONS

Following a career path in business and/or communications has generally been considered a nontraditional choice for dietitians. The Academy of Nutrition and Dietetics membership survey in 2015 indicated that about 32 percent of dietitians work in the for-profit sector, including those in contract food management, managed care organizations, and other for-profit organizations. Thirty nine percent worked in nonprofit organizations and 20 percent for governments.[2] The for-profit category also represents a wide range of positions, including private practice, owning a business, and working with corporations, trade associations, food and pharmaceutical companies, and hotels and restaurants. Private practice in clinical dietetics and nutrition is also moving to negotiated contracts with medical specialty clinics, medical departments (i.e., pediatrics, gastroenterology, internal medicine, oncology, etc.) within the hospital setting, especially as hospital stays become shorter and fewer professionals are employed on staff.

Expanded opportunities in business and communications are expected to continue and grow as employers add dietitians to their organization by realizing their value to the business. The major reasons appear to be to increase the company's credibility, to promote customer health and nutrition, and to increase the understanding of customer/consumer needs. Given the current trends reported by the Food Marketing Institute, consumers believe the main payoffs of good health are being more active, relieving stress, lowering disease risk, having more energy and living longer.[3] Food producers, food retailers, and food service establishments take note of what is important to the public and respond by providing products that help meet nutritional and other needs. Food labeling laws, healthy vending programs, the government farm bill, food safety regulations, and other governmental initiatives are helping to position good nutrition within closer reach of people.

Career Opportunities

There are many paths to a career in business and communications for interested and qualified dietitians. The importance of early exposure to the business world is increasingly recognized, as pointed out in recommendations that dietetics students experience a rotation in a business environment as part of their undergraduate study, dietetic internship, or graduate study.[4] Students and supervisors can discover opportunities by contacting exhibitors at professional meetings, local businesses, or by contacting other professionals in business and communications. A business rotation may also offer the opportunity for exposure to marketing and public relations activities that are essential in business.

The Dietitians in Business and Communications practice group identifies its members as presidents, vice presidents, food service directors, food stylists, researchers, consultants, sales managers, marketing managers, in store workshop providers, restaurateurs, test kitchen managers, and software specialists. Emerging areas involve personal/individual grocery shoppers, in-home nutrition coaches, and gourmet food preparation instruction.[5]

How does an individual get a start in business? Several steps are important, including the following:

- Make a list of your talents, skills, and interests.
- Make a list of all the possible areas in which you could work, including, but not limited to writing, speaking, publishing, research, marketing, teaching, sales, media, cooking demonstrations, counseling, coaching, managing, catering, and product development.
- Make a list of the group with whom you enjoy working and/or in which you have had some experience.
- Read journals and newsletters: the *Journal of the Academy of Nutrition and Dietetics*, Food and Nutrition magazine, dietetic practice group newsletters, and others and make a list of dietitians doing things you would enjoy doing and can do.
- Contact others working in your areas of interest—find a mentor.
- Network, network, network—with other dietitian nutritionists and professionals in related areas of practice.[6–8]

Dietitians in business and communications cite several positive things they like about their jobs: challenging work, learning opportunities, creativity, fast pace, flexible scheduling, visibility, and remuneration. At the same time, some indicate there can be stress, long hours, a fast pace, bureaucracy, a lot of information to absorb, and a critical responsibility for targeted continuing education. The dietitian who is flexible, willing to take risks, and is interested in the business world is most likely to succeed.

Mentors and Networks

The dietitian/nutritionists following nontraditional paths agree that having a mentor, networking, developing a strategic skill set, and keeping current with research and consumer trends are factors necessary to build successful careers.[9–11] A mentor may be a coworker, an instructor, or another professional. A mentor in the same organization can provide insight into policies, procedures, and the unspoken policies of a company.

Networking both inside and outside the boundaries of dietetics is a way of finding a mentor, gathering information, and connecting with others.[12] The networking offered through dietetic practice groups is invaluable to professionals looking for opportunities for change or advancement in nontraditional areas. Affiliating with other professional associations will provide more ideas and contacts. Social media (Facebook, Twitter, blogs, etc.) and technology are also involved in the communications skills needed to progress. Many otherwise traditional encounters now take place on email and social media outlets.

Strategic Skill Building

The ability to communicate effectively, along with business know-how and public relations, or people skills, is strategic to a successful career. Industry studies routinely point out that communicating well means the difference between success and failure. The ability to build on earlier education and experience leads to professional growth and enhanced job performance. For example, if a job requires evaluating research and working with research and development, a good grounding in science is important. Clinical education and experience help a dietitian nutritionist understand the health and nutritional implications when producing and marketing a new food, dietary supplement, or educational materials.

Advancing into positions with increasing responsibility and managerial skill necessitates continuing education, often in the business-related areas of study. The growth of online and distance education helps make this possible even for the professional working full time or in locations away from the educational setting. Dietitians in business frequently continue their education by acquiring an MBA or an advanced degree in management or finance.

In today's world it is imperative to establish a website and participate in social media in order for dietetic professionals to enhance their business image, complement business advertising, attract new client or customers outside the local area, or to start a new business venture.[13] They may also find this a useful way to learn more about specific businesses and to build and enhance networks.

THE DIETITIAN IN HEALTH AND WELLNESS PROGRAMS

Wellness, health promotion, corporate fitness, elite professional athletes, and sports nutrition programs are all career opportunities that have increased in recent years. Although sports and dietetics as professions or areas of interest have existed for centuries, the combination of the two as a career specialty is relatively recent. The growth of wellness and fitness programs has been rapid as the relationship between nutritional status and maintenance of health, prevention of disease, and the slowing of aging effects becomes more evident.[14]

A poor diet is a known risk factor for the development of the three chronic diseases that are the leading cause of death in adults in the United States, that is, cancer, cardiovascular disease, and stroke.[15] Additional health problems of adults are also closely associated with diet and eating behaviors, such as obesity, diabetes, high blood pressure, and osteoporosis. The number of deaths and medical costs can be significantly altered by changes in diet and lifestyle when it is considered that billions of dollars are spent each year on schemes and unproven methods to reduce body weight and prevent cancer, not to mention the money spent treating adults with these diseases and their complications.

Reports from the National Health and Nutrition Examination Survey III (NHANES) indicate an alarming increase in the prevalence and severity of obesity in young children, older children, and adolescents, as well as adults.[16] These statistics point to the need for programs in health promotion, wellness, fitness, and the prevention and treatment of obesity, all of which greatly expands career options for dietitian nutritionists.

Some dietitians have developed their own programs through practice and research and now market or license the programs to other dietitians and health professionals, both nationally and internationally. Others continue to work in hospitals, ambulatory care centers, clinics, senior living centers, rehabilitation centers, and athletic clubs or gyms. Those in private practice provide counseling and medical nutrition therapies aimed at preventing and treating obesity and other disease conditions.

Even with, or perhaps because of the increasing prevalence of obesity, many dietary fads, drugs, and questionable dieting programs have escalated and now account for enormous amounts of money each year. This phenomenon emphasizes the need and opportunities that exist for dietitians and other health professionals in this area.

Sports Nutrition

Interest in sports and cardiovascular nutrition among members of the Academy led to the formation of the Sports, Cardiovascular, and Wellness Nutrition dietetic practice group. Disordered eating as an area of practice was added to the group to include dietary professionals with an interest in this area (such as anorexia nervosa and bulimia), as they recognized the frequent presence of eating disorders among athletes and the critical role that the identification and treatment of disordered eating has in maintaining health and wellness.

The Academy of Nutrition and Dietetics, the Dietitians of Canada and the American College of Sports Nutrition issued a position paper in 2009 concerning nutrition and athletic performance.[17] The importance of optimal nutrition and the roles and responsibilities of healthcare professionals was discussed in the paper. The educational needs of those aspiring to become a sports nutritionist were detailed in an article by Clark.[18] Knowledge of nutrition and exercise science, physiology, business skills, and a foundation of strong clinical experience are all important, especially because many sports nutritionists are entrepreneurs. A list of the clinical concerns commonly presented to a sports nutritionist is shown in **Table 11-1**.

Table 11-1. Clinical Concerns Commonly Presented to a Sports Nutritionist

Allergies	Diarrhea
Alcohol addiction	Gastric reflux
Amenorrhea	Gout
Anemia	Headaches
Anorexia	Hypoglycemia
Arteriosclerosis	Hyperlipidemia
Binge eating	Hypertension
Body image distortion	Menopause
Bulimia	Obesity/overweight
Cancer (prevention, recovery form)	Osteoporosis
Chronic fatigue	Pregnancy/perinatal nutrition
Constipation	Stress fractures
Diabetes	Surgery (special nutritional pre- and postoperative)

Data from *Journal of the American Dietetic Association* 100, Number 12 (December 2000), Clark, N. "Identifying the Educational Needs of Aspiring Sports Nutritionists," 1522–1524, Copyright 2000.

Dietetic professionals with a specialty in sports nutrition can be found in a wide variety of settings, from sports medicine, rehabilitation clinics to professional athletic teams, high school athletics, the Olympics, and from colleges and universities to fitness centers, private clubs, and corporate fitness programs. Many incorporate sports nutrition into their more general practice of nutrition counseling or private practice. Today, several professional sports teams include dietitians as paid consultants whose expertise serves to enhance the player's performance. A few professional athletes have employed personal dietitians primarily to help them maintain appropriate body weight and ratio of fat to lean body mass.

Some dietitians specialize as nutrition trainers for college athletes and teams in the sport or sports in which they have the greatest personal interest, such as swimming, wrestling, baseball, or cycling.

Many dietetic professionals working in the area of sports nutrition also work as clinical dietitians for acute care facilities, as outpatient dietitians, or in private practice in nutrition counseling. In addition, some dietitians are employed to supervise the food production and training tables in college athletic residence halls. Some professional athletes seek information on diet during the off-season to maintain body weight and strength. As part of his or her daily routine, a sports nutritionist may counsel athletes one on one regarding their food intake and appropriate nutrients or their use of dietary supplemental aids.[19] A nutritionist may also conduct group classes on low-fat eating at a fitness center or work with a high school team to suggest healthful choices for eating when the team travels. Sports nutritionists also serve as part-time staff at health clubs and are available to answer questions members may ask on nutrition or to conduct classes on eating for competition and good health.

An additional career for some dietitians with experience in sports nutrition and fitness has emerged in writing and developing nutrition education materials appropriate for athletes of all ages. Other dietitians enjoy speaking and/or writing for the media and consultative arrangements with any number of organizations. Another career option that is growing emanates from the proliferation of gymnasiums and physical fitness centers for young children and adolescents. Although these gyms and centers were started for tumbling and gymnastic opportunities, there is a need for expertise in nutrition in these settings, especially combined with principles of child development. Parents and consumers are welcoming the dietitian's expertise related to treatment of obesity, weight maintenance, and disordered eating patterns in young children and adolescents. In some instances, entrepreneurial dietitians are developing centers and mobile units that go to elementary schools or other sites for demonstrations of appropriate physical activity and the benefits of good food choices and nutrition. Last but not least are the opportunities for "coaching"/ counseling family sports enthusiasts which include marathon and other competitive events for the entire family.

Knowledge of exercise physiology through course work in exercise science is essential if the sports nutritionist combines nutrition and exercise in work with clients. Many dietetic professionals work to enhance their education and expertise by entering graduate programs in exercise physiology, counseling, psychology, or business administration. In addition, although few college or university programs in sports nutrition currently exist, many graduate students choose to conduct research for their thesis or dissertation on a topic directly related to sports nutrition. By acquiring a strong foundation in foods and normal and clinical nutrition with study in a related area, the dietetic student can better prepare him or herself for practice in sports nutrition.

A list of roles and responsibilities for the sports dietitian is found in the position paper: "Position of the American Dietetic Association, Dietitians of Canada, and the American College of Sports Medicine."[20]

Cardiovascular Nutrition

With the abundance of continuing research in the area of diet and heart disease as well as the fact that heart disease remains the number one cause of death for Americans, careers in cardiovascular nutrition offer many options. Most acute-care facilities whose services include open-heart surgery have cardiac rehabilitation programs in place. These typically include inpatient and outpatient components, both of which offer nutrition counseling and education as part of the program. Cardiac rehabilitation programs include multidisciplinary teams who deal with all aspects of risk factor reduction, as well as education of the patient and family. Team members may include a medical director, cardiac rehabilitation nurse clinicians, exercise therapist, social worker, occupational therapist, and a dietitian/nutritionist. Education of the patient and family is often conducted in a variety of ways, from individual instruction to group or online classes. The dietitian may also design and conduct classes on low-fat cooking and other food preparation techniques.

Dietitians who specialize in cardiovascular nutrition may be employed by lipid research clinics. These professionals are responsible for teaching clinic patients how to change their eating habits to lower total fat and saturated fat or to comply with a research feeding protocol. In this setting as at a university, they may conduct research on the latest cardiology/nutrition methodologies. Opportunities also exist with pharmaceutical companies as sales representatives or in the public relations departments of large food companies that market products to patients with cardiovascular disease and their families.

Wellness and Health Promotion

The opportunities for dietitians in wellness and health promotion are numerous and diverse. Dietitians who specialize in wellness may have a private practice or consulting business and negotiate contracts with industry, corporations, or health clubs. Others are employed by medical centers or corporations to manage their on-site-wellness and health promotion programs, which may include conducting classes for employees, developing incentives to foster a greater interest in exercise and nutrition, and increasing productivity by helping to reduce employee illness. Because nutrition is part of wellness, dietitians specializing in wellness and health promotion may also be involved inn programs on smoking cessation, meditation and yoga, stress management, exercise, back safety, and employee relations.

Corporations and large institutions initially began providing work-site wellness programs for their employees because research and reports showed that these programs improved employee health, increased productivity, and decreased absenteeism and lost work days due to illness. As these programs developed and increased in number across the country in businesses of all sizes, data began to accumulate on the economic benefits of work-site wellness programs. With healthcare costs soaring and major changes occurring in healthcare and insurance coverage, employers were eager to explore wellness and health promotion programs that would save the corporation money. The common method for defining economic benefits is through cost-benefit ratios in which the cost is the actual dollar cost of providing the program, and benefits are expressed in dollars saved from reduced absenteeism, disability expenses, and medical costs.

The ability to work as a facilitator and to conduct classes in a group setting is an important characteristic of the successful wellness professional.

Counseling skills are also necessary because dealing with high-risk persons may be a regular aspect of the job. In addition, the dietitian must be prepared to analyze and evaluate enormous amounts of information available to employees and clients through media routes. This counseling may take place in groups, individually, at health fairs, over the telephone, or via computers.

Wellness and fitness programs are also emerging for increasing numbers in the aging and retired population as well as the younger employed groups. Research indicates that even though aging is inevitable, biologic aging can be delayed through appropriate nutrition and exercise.[21] As the number of senior citizens increases, this provides another career opportunity for dietitians specializing in health promotion as senior citizens strive to maximize independence and well-being. Programs to improve fitness and the quality of life and encourage wellness in this age group including nutrition, exercise, and lifestyle changes are developing. As most of these programs are built around a "social" model rather than a "medical" model, other professionals and non-professionals are moving to secure positions in these areas. This means that dietitian nutritionists must be proactive in promoting the unique and appropriate expertise of the dietetic professionals.

Several national organizations provide excellent and accurate information for dietitians seeking up-to-date knowledge on wellness and health promotion programs and concepts. In addition, all have information on the Internet. The major organizations with this information are the following:

- The Academy of Nutrition and Dietetics (www.eatright.org)
- International Food Information Council (www.ific.org)
- National Institutes of Health (www.nih.gov)
- Centers for Disease Control and Prevention (www.cdc.gov)
- American College of Sports Medicine (www.ascm.org)
- American Alliance on Health, Physical Education, Recreation, and Dance (www.aahperd.org)
- Food and Nutrition Information Center (www.fnic.nal.usda.gov)
- National Administration on Aging (www.aoa.acl.gov)
- American Association of Retired Persons (www.aarp.org)
- Center for Nutrition Policy and Promotion (www.cnpp.usda.gov)
- American Public Health Association (www.apha.org)

The Internet also offers the opportunity and challenge for the individual dietitian nutritionist to develop websites and disseminate nutrition and fitness messages by this means.

Disordered Eating

Dietitians who specialize in disordered eating work in a variety of settings, including residential treatment centers, hospitals (both medical and psychiatric), outpatient clinics, managed care organizations, university health centers, and private practice. The specialty of disordered or problematic eating encompasses several areas in which nutritional, physical, and psychological issues are intertwined with eating behavior, such as obesity, chronic dieting, and binge eating disorder. Complications of these disorders are potentially life threatening. Many have their origin or manifestation in childhood or adolescence. Although most of these disorders affect adolescent females, there are reports of similar behavior in males. Effective treatment of disordered eating requires knowledge and skill in counseling, cognitive behavioral therapy, family systems theory addiction, and pharmacology.[22]

Because of the biopsychological nature of disordered eating, the role of the dietitian on the treatment team is vital. The dietitian educates the client about food, physical activity, and body shape and size, and guides his or her in developing a sound eating style and physical activity pattern. Clients may share their thoughts and feeling about food, weight, and physical activity with the dietitian. They may also share life situations and events that are stressful for them, such as job change, marital problems, school problem, relationships, and burnout. The dietitian helps clients identify how stress affects their eating style and how they feel about food, their body size and shape, and physical activity. Ongoing communication with the treatment team therapist, psychiatrist, and physician is essential so that the dietitian can discern which issues are nutrition-related and which are psychological or medical. It takes years of experience for the dietitian to most effectively complement his or her skills and expertise with other members of the team.

Dietitians working in programs to treat disordered eating benefit from regular supervision from a mental health professional who specializes in problematic eating. This relationship provides a forum for discussion of specific cases, as well as helps to clarify which issues are appropriately addressed in nutrition therapy versus psychotherapy. Furthermore, many dietitians seek continuing education in areas such as women's issues, cognitive behavioral therapy, family counseling, psychotherapeutic counseling skills, and psychopharmacology. The intention is to sharpen counseling skills and enhance the understanding of sociological and psychological aspects of disordered eating while consistently staying within the scope of practice of the dietetic professional, adhering to the standards of practice and professional performance and the Academy's code of ethics.[23,24]

PRACTICE GROUPS

Dietitians in business typically join the Dietitians in Business and Communications practice group, the Management in Food and Nutrition Systems practice group, the Food and Culinary Professionals practice group, and the Nutrition Entrepreneurs practice group. By joining one or more of the groups, members are able to benefit from networking, mentoring, information exchange, professional enhancement, and leadership opportunities. The Academy practice groups have individual websites and offer their members continuing education programs, periodic newsletters, forums for exploring practice issues, and innovative products and services. In addition, the Academy code of ethics, appropriate standards of practice, and standards of professional performance provide guidance and information about practice content, ethics, and what is expected of dietetic professionals in these areas of practice.[25-27] Dietitians in health and wellness programs have a number of choices among the various clinical groups, with the Sports, Cardiovascular, and Wellness Nutrition group likely the primary choice. Others are Behavioral Health Nutrition and Weight Management. Standards of practice and professional performance are available for these areas as well.[28-32]

SUMMARY

The dietitian in business and communications often deals with the public in visible and varied ways. The opportunities in these areas continually expand as consumers, employers, and government authorities become increasingly aware of the health benefits of good food choices and seek valid information.

Dietitians with expertise in worksite wellness, sports and cardiovascular nutrition, and disordered eating are increasingly in demand in nontraditional settings. They must be creative, proactive, and adept in the promotion of healthy eating behaviors and the unique expertise of the dietitian nutritionist. In addition, nutrition information and education must be presented in a manner that is directly usable by consumers. The dietitian nutritionist must be able to translate scientific information into user-friendly terms that distinguish between fact and fiction for consumers.

DEFINITIONS

Anorexia nervosa. An eating disorder characterized by a preoccupation with dieting and thinness that leads to excessive weight loss.

Bulimia nervosa. An eating disorder involving frequent episodes of binge eating followed by purging, also leading to excessive weight loss.

Cardiovascular nutrition. Application of medical nutrition therapy for those with heart and blood vessel conditions or to prevent the diseases.

Disordered eating. Abnormal eating patterns.

Health promotion. Education and preventive measures directed toward healthy populations to foster wellness and prevention of disease.

Networking. Activities directed toward making connections with others through varied contacts.

Sports nutrition. The area of nutrition specific to the needs of those who participate in sports activities.

Wellness. State of optimal health and the absence of disease.

REFERENCES

1. Simopoulos, A. "A Declaration of Olympia on Nutrition and Fitness." *Nutr Today* 3 (1996): 250–252.
2. Rogers, D. "Compensation and Benefits Survey 2015," *J Acad Nutr Diet* 116, no. 3 (2016): 370–388.
3. Food Marketing Institute. "Trends in the United States: Consumer Attitudes and the Supermarket." www.fmi.org
4. Kapica, C, and J.O.S. Maillet. "A Business Rotation for Dietitians—An Imperative in the New Millennium." *J Am Diet Assoc* 102 (2002): 1220.

5. Indorato, D.A. "Innovative Services by and for the Dietitian." *Today's Dietitian* 3 (2001): 16–19.

6. Eliot, K.A., and K.M. Kolasa. "The Value in Interprofessional, Collaborative-ready nutrition, and Dietetics practitioners." *J Acad Nutr Diet* 115, no. 10 (2015): 1578–1588.

7. DiMaria-Ghalili, R.A., J.M. Murtallo, B.W. Tobin, L. Hark, L. Van Horn, and C.A. Palmer. "Challenges and Opportunities for Nutrition Education and Training in the Health Care Professions: Intraprofessional and Interprofessional Call to Action." *Am J Clin Nutr* 99, suppl 5 (2014): 1184S–1193S.

8. Institute of Medicine. *Building Health Workforce Capacity through Community-based Health Professional Education.* Workshop Summary. (Washington, DC: The National Academies Press: October 3, 2014). www.iom.edu/reports/2014/BuildingHealthWorkforceCapaity. (4/28/2016).

9. Academy of Nutrition and Dietetics, www.eatrightpro.org/public/page

10. Lipscomb, R., and S. An. "Mentoring 101: Building a Mentoring Relationship." *J Acad Nutr Diet* 113, no. 5 (2013): S29–S31.

11. Peregrin, T. "Mentoring Can Be An Effective Professional Development Experience to Enhance or Expand Your Career." *J Acad Nutr Diet* 113, no. 5 (2013): S42–S47.

12. See Note 6.

13. Pangan, T, and C. Bedner. "Dietitian Business Websites: A survey of Their Profitability and How You Can Make Yours Profitable. *J Am Diet Assoc* 102 (2002): 399–402.

14. Golson, S.K. "Make Time for Daily Physical Activity." *J Am Diet Assoc* 109 (2009): 18.

15. National Center for Health Statistics. "Data 1997–2010." www.cdc.gov

16. Centers for Disease Control and Prevention. "Overweight among Children and Adolescents, 16–19 Years of Age, by Selected Characteristics. U.S. 963–65 through 2005–2006." www.cdc.gov

17. Nutrition and Athletic Performance for Adults. "Position of the Academy of Nutrition and Dietetics, Dietitians of Canada, and the American College of Sports Medicine: Nutrition and Athletic Performance." *J Am Diet Assoc* 116 (2016): 509–527.

18. Clark, N. "Identifying the Educational Needs of Aspiring Sports Nutritionists." *J Am Diet Assoc* 100 (2000): 1522–1524.

19. Shattuck, D. "Sports Nutritionists Feel the Competitive Edge." *J Am Diet Assoc* 101 (2001): 517–518.

20. See Note 17.

21. Etgen, T., D. Sander, U. Huntgeburth, H. Pappas, H. Fasti, and H. Bickel. "Physical Activity and Incident Cognitive Impairment in Elderly Persons." *Arch Intern Med* 170 (2010): 186–193.

22. Nutrition Intervention in the Treatment of Eating Disorders. Position Paper. *J Am Diet Assoc* 2011;111:1236–1241.

23. Tholking, M.M., A.C. Mellowsprings, S.G. Eberle, R.P. Lamb, E.S. Myers, C.S. Scribner, R.F. Sloan, et al. "American Dietetic Association: Standards of Practice and Standards of Professional Performance for Registered (Competent, Proficient, and Expert) in Disordered Eating Disorders (DE and Ed)." *J Am Diet Assoc* 111 (2011): 1241–1249.

24. American Dietetic Association/Commission on Dietetic Registration. "Code of Ethics for the Profession of Dietetics and Process for Consideration of Ethics Issues." *J Am Diet Assoc* 109 (2009): 1461–1467.

25. See Note 24.

26. Academy of Nutrition and Dietetics Quality Management Committee and Scope of Practice Subcommittee of the Quality Management Committee. "Revised 2012 Standards of Practice in Nutrition Care and Standards of Professional Performance for Registered Dietitians." *J Acad Nutr Diet* 113, no. 6 (2013): S29–S45.

27. Academy of Nutrition and Dietetics Quality Management Committee and Scope of Practice Subcommittee of the Quality Management Committee. "Revised 2012 Standards of Practice in Nutrition Care and Standards of Professional Performance for Dietetic Technicians, Registered." *J Acad Nutr Diet* 113 (2013): S56–S71.

28. Academy of Nutrition and Dietetics Quality Management Committee and Scope of Practice Subcommittee of the Quality Management Committee. "Scope of Practice for the Registered Dietitian." *J Acad Nutr Diet* 113, no. 6 (2013): S17–S28.

29. Academy of Nutrition and Dietetics Quality Management Committee and Scope of Practice Subcommittee of the Quality Management Committee. "Scope of Practice for the Dietetic Technician, Registered." *J Acad Nutr Diet* 113, no. 6 (2013): S46–S55.

30. Steinmuller, P.L., L.J. Kruskall, C.A. Karpinski, M.M. Manore, M.A. Macedonia, N.L. Meyer. "Academy of Nutrition and Dietetics. Revised 2014 Standards of Practice and Standards of Professional Performance for Registered Dietitian Nutritionists (Competent, Proficient, and Expert) in Sports Nutrition and Dietetics." *J Acad Nutr Diet* 114 (2014): 631–641.

31. Emerson, M.P., P. Kerr, M.D.C. Soler, T.A. Girard, R. Hofflinger, E. Pritchett, and M. Otto. "American Dietetic Association Standards of Practice and Standards of Professional Performance for Registered Dietitians (Generalist, Specialty, and Advanced) in Behavioral Health Care." *J Am Diet Assoc* 106 (2006): 608–613.

32. Jortberg, B., F. Myers, L. Gigliotti, B.J. Ivens, M. Lebre, S.B. March, I. Nogueira, et al. "Academy of Nutrition and Dietetics: Standards of Practice and Standards of Professional Performance for Registered Dietitian Nutritionists (Competent, Proficient, and Expert) in Adult Weight Management." *J Acad Nutr Diet* 115, no. 4 (2015): 609–618.

CHAPTER 12

The Dietitian as Manager and Leader

"Skills such as team building, delegation, communication, negotiation, and self-management are fundamental to high performance. Fortunately, these can be learned and enhanced through continuing education and training."[1]

OUTLINE

LEARNING OBJECTIVES

The student will be able to:

1. Become aware of the characteristics of leaders and managers.
2. Become familiar with how leadership skill is attained.
3. Understand how leadership skills contribute to quality and efficiency in an organization.
4. Understand the interrelationship between technical, human relations, and conceptual skills in management.
5. Explain the importance of management skill in clinical and community practice.

INTRODUCTION

Management is often regarded as the responsibilities and challenges that have to do with being in charge or being the boss of a department, and therefore, the entry-level dietitian often believes that he or she does not need to be concerned with knowing how to manage. In reality, all dietitians, regardless of their job title or job responsibilities, perform many managerial functions and need to develop managerial skills. The clinical dietitian, the food service manager, the nutritionist in community nutrition programs, the educator, the private practitioner, the dietitian in business and industry, and healthcare administrators all perform management functions. Among these functions are setting goals, evaluating outcomes, managing resources, integrating and coordinating personnel activities, training personnel and allied professionals, communicating, and promoting quality control.

Management and leadership have many overlapping characteristics and have been described in several ways by leaders in the management field. A simplified way to view them is to think of management as the activities that go into making a department or an institution run—doing things—and leadership as the qualities a person (a manager) needs to possess in order to make things go right. We could say "things are managed and people are led."[2]

In this chapter, we discuss leadership and management separately, but because many functions are complementary, both need to be developed together. A professional cannot be truly successful unless characteristics of both leadership and management skills are evident in the workplace.

LEADERSHIP

Frank[3] describes leadership as "the art of bringing together people with diverse talents, interests, ideas, and backgrounds to voluntarily participate in a shared approach toward common or compatible goals." This definition makes the distinction between accomplishing tasks and inspiring people to willingly perform those tasks. Leadership consists of the traits that accompany good management skills, and for someone to be successful, the two functions need to go together.

Leaders and thinkers, including Peter Drucker, who is recognized as an authority on leadership, consider that three important characteristics for successful leadership are:[4]

1. Thinking through the mission of the organization, defining it, and establishing it clearly and visibly. The leader sets the goals and priorities and maintains the standards.
2. Viewing leadership as a responsibility and not a rank or a privilege. Effective leaders are rarely permissive, but when things go wrong, they do not blame others. They encourage and help develop strong associates.
3. Earning trust in order to have followers. To trust a leader, it is not necessary to like or to agree; rather trust is the conviction that the leader means what he or she says and has integrity.

Attaining Leadership Skills

A question often debated is whether people are born leaders or whether they develop leadership skills and thereby become leaders. In support of the view that leadership skills can be acquired, several actions that make for leadership development are the following:[5]

- Well-defined values
- Commitment to quality
- Responsive to the consumer, client, and the public
- Stimulating a nurturing work environment
- Creativity and innovation
- Open lines of communication and shared information
- Inclusive process for decision making
- Planning and fostering meaningful change to achieve goals and improved performance

Leadership Development

The American Dietetic Association (ADA) developed the Institute for Leadership in 2003.[6] At a yearly event, members received training in leadership, dialogue, and sharing perspectives through private, personalized agendas. Interactive breakout sessions and workshops as well as structured networking events were a part of the annual sessions. A certificate of training is offered at the conclusion of each annual forum. The institute was discontinued in 2011. Now, however, the Academy offers an online leadership certificate program, offering two levels of leadership training. The level 2 program, introduced in 2014, offers four modules of learning.[7]

In reviewing traditional leadership theory, it has been suggested that more information is needed about the way dietitians develop as leaders.[8] Consistent with earlier theories about the way humans grow through stages of mental development and become leaders in predictable ways, a newer theory is that of constructive development, described as an alternative approach to leadership as a way of growing in stages.[9] Studies of leaders across industries and organizational levels show that 5 percent of all leaders are at a stage where they are focused on self and seldom welcome feedback; 80 percent are in a middle stage of avoiding conflict, becoming a member of a group, having a strong belief system, and being result and goal oriented, while 15 percent are at the highest stage during which there is systematic problem solving, seeking feedback, realizing the complexity of the environment, and having a deep appreciation of others. When a survey of Academy leaders was conducted in 2006, most were shown to be in the high part of the medium range group. It is suggested that by becoming aware of their own stage, dietitians can develop further in their leadership ability by seeking out a supportive environment, perhaps through advanced study, mentors, supportive coworkers, networking, and others.

Another aspect of leadership is the need for what has become known as emotional intelligence, along with intellectual and technical skills. The most effective leader has a high degree of emotional intelligence. This is defined as self-awareness, self-regulation, motivation, empathy, and social skills. These skills can be learned through experience and internal commitment.[10]

Leadership for Quality and Efficiency

Leadership development programs, increasingly conducted in hospitals and other healthcare organizations, improve both the quality and efficiency of care. Opportunities found to result from four qualitative studies of leadership development are the following:[11]

- Improve the quality of the workforce
- Increase efficiency in the organization's education and development activities
- Reduce turnover and related expenses
- Focus organizational attention on specific priorities

MANAGEMENT FUNCTIONS

Management is usually defined in terms of the traditional functions described by management experts. Although the number of functions varies according to the way in which they are presented, the following six are universally accepted:[12]

1. *Planning.* Planning is the activity of setting goals and objectives. The extent of the planning, from setting broad, long-range goals for a large organization to planning shorter term goals, will usually be determined by where persons are in the organizational hierarchy.
2. *Organizing.* Organizing is the reflection of how the organization accomplishes its goals and objectives. The tasks to be performed, assignment of tasks, allocation of resources, and flow of authority and communication are established.
3. *Coordinating.* Coordinating involves activities that lead to the efficient use of resources to attain the goals and objectives.
4. *Staffing.* Staffing means determining human resource needs, then recruiting, selecting, hiring, and training the necessary staff.
5. *Directing.* Directing (or leading) refers to those activities that enable accomplishment of the organization goals, that communicate those goals, and that create an atmosphere that encourages commitment and desired performance.
6. *Controlling.* Controlling occurs when performance is assessed against standards that have been translated from the goals and objectives and corrective measures applied as needed.

Dietitians who are experienced in management areas of practice are aware that overarching all those activities is the need to communicate effectively—realizing that this is always a two-way process—and to develop the ability to work in productive ways with others in the organization at all levels. Setting goals and standards, incorporating as much technology as feasible and needed, and being financially astute are all critical to successful practice.

SKILLS AND ABILITIES OF MANAGERS

Three fundamental sets of skills needed by managers at various levels to function effectively are human relations skills, technical skills, and conceptual skills (**Figure 12-1**). Earlier traditional views of management held that top managers primarily needed human relations and conceptual skills, while the more contemporary view is that technical skills as well are increasingly important for the top manager, especially in small organizations and in those with flattened and decentralized organizational patterns. What is immediately apparent from Figure 12-1 is that all levels of managers and even employees need to possess equal amounts of human

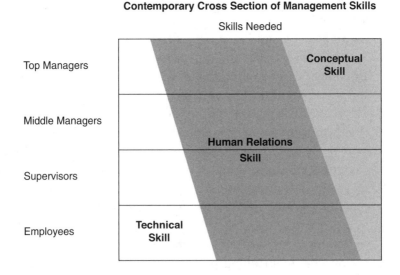

FIGURE 12-1. Balancing Management and Leadership.

Reproduced from Woods RH, King JZ. Leadership and Management in the Hospitality Industry. 3rd ed. Lansing, MI. American Hotel and Lodging Educational Institute, 2010, p. 56.

relations skills that are predominant among the three sets of skills. The need for technical skills increases with lesser overall managerial responsibilities, while the higher conceptual skills decrease. The use of particular skills, such as the need to hire and train new employees or to engage in long-range strategic planning, will vary from day to day with changes in the work environment. The specific activities practiced in these three skill areas are discussed in the following sections.

Human Relations Skills

Interpersonal Relationships

Interpersonal skills are always rated highly when management skills are described or studied. The ability to work with others toward common goals is the number one factor denoting success among healthcare departmental managers.[13] Human factors may also influence how this is done successfully; for instance, regulatory requirements such as the Family Medical Leave Act (FMLA) provide job security for workers but may also present labor coverage problems for the manager. Changing job assignments, paying overtime, or bringing additional workers can affect resources and make the manager's job more difficult.

Generational diversity, or the involvement of several distinct generations in the workplace, presents another aspect of achieving successful working relationships.[14] Different generations of workers are assumed to have different loyalties and expectations resulting in the need for open-mindedness, effective communication, and respect for others on the part of the manager. Dealing with language skills, literacy, and other sociocultural issues can impact relationships.[15]

Communication

Communication at both individual and group levels ensures that information flow reaches all those in an organization. Keeping others informed, seeking input from others in the organization, and rewarding staff for good work and successes lead to satisfaction and cooperation. Staff members are excellent sources of information, ideas, and solutions, and should always be involved when new programs or procedures are being planned. The manager needs to receive information from as many sources as possible and no one in the organization should be overlooked for this input.

The skillful communicator is often one who is also a transformational leader. Such a manager stimulates innovative ways of thinking, can achieve greater performance on the part of those managed and has vision that can lead to organizational change when needed. By communicating openly and directly with all members of a team, others are motivated to share in commitment to the needs of the group as a whole.[16]

Coaching and Mentoring

Most dietitians will be, at some time in their career, in the position of assisting and supporting a coworker or employee as they learn a new job or develop new skills, and thus will become a coach or mentor. A mentor is described as a person who teaches through verbal instruction, demonstration of particular activities or skills, and role modeling. Coaching is similar in that it is used to inspire and motivate as well as teach. The successful dietitian may function in both these roles in order to accomplish needed tasks. Staff personnel perform at different levels and learn in different ways. It is the enterprising coach or mentor who is able to adapt actions to motivate, encourage, and support staff, thereby creating a productive and harmonious team. Mentoring is discussed in greater detail later in this text.

Managing Conflict

Conflict occurs in any organization and wherever people work in groups. Conflict may arise from competition for resources, overlapping responsibilities, status struggles, poor communications, inadequate training, or differences in values and beliefs. The dietitian who recognizes causes of conflict and assists in taking steps to overcome the differences will be looked to as a manager and leader. When dealt with quickly and constructively, conflict can be a way of improving performance.[17]

Networking

Networking within an organization leads to both communication and cooperation. People form networks for sharing social and business information and to increase professional competence. Sharing information is vital in any organization, and the manager will seek opportunities to network both within and beyond the work unit and will encourage others to also network. Networking with other professionals through the dietetic practice groups of the Academy and other groups can lead to personal growth, a greater understanding of practice requirements, and enhanced performance in every area of practice.

Technical Skills

Technical skills are those that require a specialized knowledge of techniques, methods, procedures, and processes that accomplish the work of an organization. Knowing how to access and use technology for communications is a must for all professionals in the modern workplace. Online information is rapidly becoming the means by which professionals remain current. Conferences, workshops, meetings, and classes are offered online, by teleconference, or by similar means using newer technology. Not only is communications technology of increasing importance, but technology related to better and faster job performance benefits both individuals and an organization. To the extent that professionals become experts in the technology needed for their jobs, they will also become mentors and coaches for others.

Technology is used in food production and food service and in all areas of clinical practice. Computerized work schedules, purchasing and inventory control, employee records, and production schedules are examples. These activities point to the need for continual training for all staff and a strong working knowledge of the use of technical equipment of all kinds.

Job Skills

The manager has knowledge of what is required of the workforce to perform in an organization but does not generally perform the work except on an as-needed basis. However, this knowledge allows the manager to supervise those with the specific skills to fulfill the job requirements. The need to have job know-how is essential to assess performance, meet goals, and ensure quality outputs.

Resource Management

Financial management, including cost controls and budget management, comes to mind first when the management of resources is described as a management function. Resources, however, can also refer to job-related supplies and equipment, staff assistance, and even time and energy. Every dietitian and dietetic technician carries certain responsibilities for managing resources and also may be involved in budgeting and long-range planning for the use of resources.

The importance of including financial management in dietetics programs is emphasized by dietetics program directors. In one survey, educators agreed or strongly agreed with the statement, "Entry-level registered dietitians need to be trained in financial management concepts as well as clinical concepts in order to be competent practitioners."[18]

Benchmarking is a process by which the manager can measure the efficiency of work, the products produced, and the services for comparison and improvement.[19] This process is used in both healthcare and food services. Performance measures that include financial management, customer service, human resources, and operational activities are evaluated in the benchmarking process. Measurements used provide information that can be compared and used for improvement.

Training and Staff Development

The responsibility for hiring and training personnel is primarily that of upper-level management; however, all professionals will at times help train and develop new employees or other professionals. The team concept often followed in healthcare institutions, food service, and hospitality requires that all members of a team function fully and efficiently. Further, team members must know their job-related roles as well as their expected roles as a team member. Efficiency evolves from knowledge and practice and must be encouraged and assisted by those already experienced within an organization.

Team Building

A team functions in ways that support individual efforts and leads to greater productivity. Teams vary in number, may be formal or informal, and may form in a variety of ways. For instance, a team may be formed within a department or from several departments or disciplines to accomplish more than can be accomplished by individuals. Teams may also be temporary or permanent.

The value of teams lies in sharing knowledge and working toward common goals using the experience and expertise of several people in decision making and problem solving. The manager encourages teams and helps make them effective by arranging for persons to participate and providing for training of team members as needed. Teams function best when they are empowered with authority or legal power to reach a level of self-management.[20]

Work groups of persons working together for a common purpose are often formed. As with teams, they may be formally constituted or may function in an informal way such as a gathering of people to solve daily problems. The group leader has several tasks, which include understanding the internal workings of the group, planning ahead and being proactive, and managing interpersonal relations for group cohesion.

Quality Management

Quality is defined as meeting standards and expectations, sometimes in terms of high quality or above a norm or average. The Quality Management Committee of the Academy provides direction for monitoring, developing, approving, evaluating, and maintaining quality management in dietetics. The team members of the group interact with the Scope of Practice Framework committee, the Evidence-Based practice committee, and the Nutrition Care Process committee. Quality assurance in practice results through the coordinated efforts of these groups.

Dietitians in all areas of practice can monitor their own quality of work through the *Code of Ethics for the Profession of Dietetics,* the standards of professional performance, and the professional development portfolio. The outcome is competent practice and a basis for quality improvement.

In the 2010 Commission on Dietetic Registration practice audit,[21] 58 percent of entry-level dietitians indicated they perform quality assurance or performance management.

Every institution, department, business, or professional association strives to produce quality goods, services, and people. Rather than relying on subjective methods to detect quality, most organizations establish performance measures by which they assess and ensure continuous quality. In dietetics, performance standards are in effect and are described in other sections of this book. Food production managers use performance measures to ensure the quality of the food service. Patient satisfaction surveys are used for ongoing assessment of the services received. Clinical outcomes can be measured for quality through specific established indicators. The community nutritionist measures quality by satisfactory outcomes of persons receiving instruction and care. The educator measures outcomes and the quality of the education by how his or her students perform. Quality control is a part of every dietitian's job responsibility and is a managerial function.

Conceptual Skills

The manager performs a certain number of activities based on visualizing the larger picture beyond the technical aspects of his or her position. The ability to realistically anticipate the future, to plan and set goals, to provide direction in an organization, and to model professional behavior constitutes conceptual ability or skill.

Strategic Planning and Goal Setting

In general, strategic planning occurs at the upper levels of management as it requires data gathering and analysis; development of strategies, goals, and objectives; and implementation of action plans. However, professionals at all levels in an organization participate in data gathering and in setting short- and long-term goals. They are a part of the planning process to set direction and plans of action for the organization.

Some plans are general, such as the determination of values, mission, and vision statements. Others are more detailed and may be developed at the supervisory level. If operational plans are short range, they are usually expected to occur within a year. Long-term plans extend beyond 1 year—sometimes beyond 10 years. The food and nutrition professional often contributes to both types of planning by conducting feasibility studies, cost-effectiveness studies, and quality-control measures.

Ethical Conduct

In dietetics, the *Code of Ethics for the Profession of Dietetics* is the guiding document to ethical practice. In any institution, the manager or leader assists in developing organization practices and policies that promote ethical practice. Such practices are established in purchasing, financial management, patient care issues, and information provided by patients and clients. The manager or leader sets the example for ethical behavior and integrity built on openness and trust.

Managing Change

Change occurs when there is dissatisfaction with things as they are and there is a desire to change them. Change may occur slowly or rapidly as in the event of sudden or unplanned circumstances. The leader who welcomes change and uses it to motivate and improve a department will be the most successful. When members of a unit work together to make changes, the efforts are usually rewarded by acceptance of the new procedure by all those affected. In contrast, if change is imposed by the leader without input from the other members, there is often resistance and slow acceptance.

Dietitians who counsel clients to make changes do not always meet with success. Time constraints and client expectations as well as motivations that differ from those of the dietitian are factors in the change process. Change models that take into consideration the complexities of behavior and one's approach to what it takes to help people change are often helpful. One approach is the use of goal setting in a way that the client being counseled is a part of the process and understands the expected outcome.[22]

The first step in initiating change is identifying the problem. One or more achievable goals for overcoming the problem are set next. In acting, persons typically mobilize their personal and social resources and identify barriers to reaching the goal. Self-monitoring and rewards provide additional motivation to attain the goal. The reward may be external, but an effective internal reward is one such as learning that leads to sustained performance and further goal setting.

Dietetics professionals constantly face change because of new developments in health care, organizational change, and shifts in management with a new mission and vision goals. Even environmental and political situations create change. When changes are viewed as opportunities, they are more likely to lead to positive results. The creative manager or leader helps create an atmosphere that welcomes and plans for this outcome.

Common Competencies for Healthcare Managers

The Healthcare Leadership Alliance is a consortium of six major professional organizations.[23] A study conducted by the alliance reported on the following five competencies common among practicing healthcare managers (**Figure 12-2**):

1. *Communication and relationship management:* The ability to communicate clearly and concisely with internal and external customers and facilitate interactions with individuals and groups.
2. *Leadership:* The ability to inspire excellence, create and attain shared vision, and manage change.

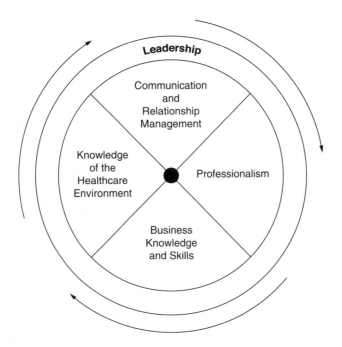

FIGURE 12-2. The Healthcare Leadership Alliance Competency Model.

3. *Professionalism:* The ability to align personal and organizational conduct with ethical and professional standards that include a responsibility to the patient and community, a service orientation, and a commitment to lifelong learning and improvement.
4. *Knowledge of the healthcare environment:* The demonstrated understanding of the healthcare system and the environment in which healthcare managers and providers function.
5. *Business skills and knowledge:* The ability to apply business principles, including systems thinking, in the healthcare environment.

MANAGEMENT IN PRACTICE

Management of food and nutrition systems is a diverse, dynamic area of practice that requires registered dietitian nutritionist (RDN) leaders who are effective in the management of human, material, and financial resources. They also need to be visionary in navigating programs and services through ever changing times in health care and other business. Public interest and healthier eating options are growing. This is in response to the obesity incidence of the population and a general interest in healthier lifestyles. Hospitals are being challenged to offer healthy food options in employee and visitor dining rooms as well as for patients.[24]

Personnel issues are without doubt one of the most time-consuming but critical parts of a manager's job. Motivating and inspiring is a large part of the job, which requires constant and effective communication, feedback on performance, and a conscious focus on cultural issues. Likewise, reviewing and updating training methods and materials can be an effective way of keeping personnel interested and motivated.

A focus on quality in every aspect of a food service system or clinical unit is a must in order to ensure acceptance by patients and clients. Even though quality is not easy to define, it is recognized—both when apparent and when lacking. The astute manager continually monitors performance of the unit by using customer surveys and informal feedback and by soliciting employee input. He or she regularly reviews all standards of ethical practice and ensures that they are fully understood and practiced by all in the organization. Ethical practices at all levels in a department create the environment in which an emphasis on quality is routine and ongoing.

The effective manager uses all available resources for continual improvement. Using the evidence-based library materials, networking with others in a practice group, and mentoring students and interns help keep the practitioner current. Further, the manager of the unit will benefit by ensuring that others in the work unit have continued education opportunities.

The management role is one that is multifaceted. It is one that requires technical know-how but just as importantly, people skills, as has been pointed out in the descriptions of managers' multiple roles.

SUMMARY

Managers and leaders possess many characteristics that are similar, but there are differences in roles and responsibilities. The skillful manager possesses human, technical, and conceptual abilities that permit him or her to accomplish work through coworkers and to attain goals. The leader may perform some or all of these same functions but will also inspire, motivate, and create a sense of unity and purpose. The dietitian, regardless of the area of practice, must perform managerial functions such as goal setting, communicating, team building, and managing resources. Many critical functions in the workplace will also require the dietitian to lead.

DEFINITIONS

Benchmarking. Comparing performance measures for the development of better methods and procedures.

Coach. A person who guides, inspires, and motivates.

Leadership. The qualities that allow an individual to influence the actions of others.

Mentor. A person who teaches and guides by instructing, demonstrating, encouraging, and role modeling.

Resource management. The handling of money, equipment and supplies, or personnel essential to the administration of an organizational unit.

Strategic planning. Long-range planning that involves data gathering, data analysis, development of goals and objectives, and action plans.

REFERENCES

1. Covey, S.R. *Principle-Centered Leadership*. (New York: Simon and Schuster, 1990).
2. Canter, D.D., K.L. Sauer, and C.W. Shanklin. "Management Is a Multifaceted Component Essential to the Skill Set of Successful Dietetics Practitioners." *J Acad Nutr Diet* 112, suppl. 2 (2012): S5.
3. Frank, G.C. *Community Nutrition: Applying Epidemiology to Contemporary Practice*. (Sudbury, MA: Jones and Bartlett, 2008).
4. Drucker, P.F. *Managing for the Future: The 1990s and Beyond*. (New York: Ruman Talley Books, Plume, 1992).
5. Cloud, H. In: M. Kaufman. *Nutrition in Promoting the Public's Health. Strategies, Principles, and Practice*. (Sudbury MA: Jones and Bartlett, 2007): 537–549.
6. Leadership Institute, 2012. www.eatright.org
7. Boyce, B. "Learning to Lead: Developing Dietetics Leaders." *J Acad Nutr Diet* 114, no. 5 (2014): 688–692.
8. Gregoire, M.B., and S.W. Arendt. "Leadership: Reflections over the Past 100 Years." *J Am Diet Assoc* 104 (2004): 395–403.

9. Hunter, A.M.B., N.M. Lewis, and P.K. Ritter-Gooder. "Constructive Developmental Theory: An Alternative Approach to Leadership." *J Am Diet Assoc* 111 (2011): 1804–1808.

10. Coleman, E. "What Makes a Leader?" *Har Bus Rev* (November–December 1998): 23–32.

11. McLearney, A.S. "Using Leadership Development Programs to Improve Quality and Efficiency in Healthcare." *J Healthcare Management* 53, no. 5 (2008): 319–331.

12. Gould, R.S., and D. Canter. "Management Matters." *J Am Diet Assoc* 108 (2008): 1834–1836.

13. Canter, D., and M.F. Nettles. "Dietitians as Multidepartment Managers in Health Care Settings." *J Am Diet Assoc* 103 (2003): 237–240.

14. Brown, D. "Ways Dietitians of Different Generations Can Work Together." *J Am Diet Assoc* 103 (2003): 1461–1462.

15. "Practice Paper of the Academy of Nutrition and Dietetics: Principles of Productivity in Food and Nutrition Services: Applications in the 21st Century Healthcare Reform Era." *J Acad Nutr Diet* 115, no. 7 (2015): 1141–1147.

16. Curtis, E.L.K., and R. O'Connell. "Essential Leadership Skills for Motivating and Developing Staff." *Nurs Manage* 18 (2011): 32–35.

17. Bartosek, C.B. In: M. Kaufman. *Nutrition in Promoting the Public Health: Strategies, Principles, and Practice.* (Sudbury, MA: Jones and Bartlett, 2007), 471.

18. McKnight, I.E.G., M.L. Dundas, and J.T. Girvan. "Dietetics Program Directors Areas of Practice." *J Am Diet Assoc* 102 (2002): 82–84.

19. Johnson, B.C., and J. Chambers. "Foodservice Benchmarking: Practices, Attitudes, and Beliefs of Foodservice Directors." *J Am Diet Assoc* 100 (2000): 175–180.

20. Weisberg, K. "Spirited Pioneer." *Foodservice Dir* 5 (2007): 65–66.

21. Ward, B.D., C. Roger, R. Mueller, R. Touger-Decker, and K.L. Sauer. "Entry-Level Dietetics Practice Today: Results from the 2010 Commission on Dietetic Registration Entry-Level Dietetics Practice Audit." *J Am Diet Assoc* 111 (2011): 914–941.

22. Cullen, K.W., T. Baranowski, and S.P. Smith. "Using Goal Setting as a Strategy for Dietary Behavior Change." *J Am Diet Assoc* 102 (2001): 562–565.

23. Steff, M.E. "Common Competencies for All Healthcare Managers: The Healthcare Leadership Alliance Model." *J Healthcare Management* 53 (2008): 360–373.

24. See Note 15.

The Dietitian as Educator

"Continuing education within the workforce must be coupled with lifelong learning to keep pace with advancements made within healthcare and technology."[1]

OUTLINE

- Learning Objectives
- Introduction
- Educational Activities of Dietitians
- Learning to Teach
- Career Opportunities in Education
  - Elementary and Secondary Schools
  - Colleges and Universities
  - Medical and Dental Education
  - Nursing and Allied Health Nutrition Education
  - Industry-Based Education
  - Work-Site Nutrition Education
- Educator Roles
  - Mentor
  - Coach
  - Preceptor
  - Counselor
  - Communicator
- Types of Learning
  - Service Learning
  - Problem-Based Learning
  - Project-Based Learning
- Adults as Learners

LEARNING OBJECTIVES

The student will be able to:
1. Discuss the steps involved in learning to teach.
2. Become familiar with career options in education.
3. Describe the mentor, coach, and preceptor role.
4. Explain how communication is a vital part of education.
5. Discuss learning styles of persons at differing age groups.
6. Give examples of a dietitian's (in any area of practice) educator role.

INTRODUCTION

Dietitians sometimes reveal that they chose dietetics as a career in part because they did not view themselves as teachers. The reality, however, is that all dietitians are educators, most frequently in locations other than the classroom. The educational settings are as diverse as the careers in which dietitians work; the learners are individuals and groups of all ages. For example, the dietitian who works in clinical dietetics in a hospital or healthcare center teaches patients, families, and allied health personnel. A dietitian in food service management teaches and trains food service personnel and may teach personnel in other departments. Dietitians in business or private practice may teach patients, other personnel, and the public. In all areas of practice, the dietitian may also teach dietetic interns and dietetic technician students.

The educator role is one of the most important a dietitian fulfills. Knowledge of subject matter is attained by the professional through academic preparation in a degree program and practical experience in a supervised practice program. Added to this knowledge is an understanding of how to teach effectively and how people learn. Observation of other educators, continuing education, and professional experience, as well as practice, lead to expertise as an educator.

Dietitians need to possess several skills related to teaching. These include verbal and nonverbal communications, speaking to groups, behavior modification and motivation, principles of learning, teaching techniques, and knowledge about how to work with groups. These skills can be learned and improved the more they are practiced.

Dietitians in education typically affiliate with one of the three following dietetic practice groups: Nutrition Education for the Public, Nutrition Educators of Health Professionals, or Dietetic Educators of Practitioners.

EDUCATIONAL ACTIVITIES OF DIETITIANS

The Commission on Dietetic Registration (CDR) periodically indicates the educational activities performed by entry-level dietitians and dietetic technicians.[2] The activities are shown in **Table 13-1**.

Table 13-1. % of Educational Activities Performed by Entry-Level Dietitians and Dietetic Technicians

Activity	RD Percent	DTR Percent
Asses Assess learning needs of patients/clients, employees, and students	90	73
Develop instructional materials for individuals and group	81	58
Teach classes or laboratories	48	38
Evaluate learner knowledge and performance	64	48
Supervise students or precept interns	55	32
Provide health-promotion or risk-reduction programs to population groups	21	12
Distribute nutrition information through the media	17	6
Design individual courses or seminars for patients, clients, employees, and students		51
Design group-related courses for educational institutions	16	0
Evaluate educational programs	23	0
Design services to meet nutrition-related needs of population	19	0

This article was published in the *Journal of the American Dietetic Association*, 92(12), Roach, et al, "Improving Dietitians' Teaching Skills," pp. 1749–1757, Copyright Elsevier (2001).

LEARNING TO TEACH

Teaching skills are developed when the educator follows a process that will result in an effective outcome; that is, the learner is a participant in the process and acquires new knowledge. Depending on the type of teaching session—formal as in a classroom or informal as in the workplace—the process may involve a very structured plan that follows specific steps or a more flexible plan with input from learners.

The steps in the process are the following:

1. The assessment of learner needs
2. The development of performance objectives
3. The instructional strategy including content and delivery method
4. Preparation of instructional materials
5. Evaluation or follow-up of the learning session

The steps may be shortened or compressed in informal teaching situations; nevertheless, thought should be given to each of the steps whether in a one-on-one session or in group sessions. In the first step, the assessment of learner needs is the basis for planning a teaching session. This may be determined from practical experience and observation of job performance, a change in organizational needs, a job change, or whether it is new information or a reinforcement of the learner's understanding of information presented earlier. Having one or more objectives in mind gives focus to the teaching session and provides a reference later as to the effectiveness of the lesson.

The content of the lesson and the way the material is to be presented require advance planning along with the determination of teaching aids needed. The content and the way it is presented can vary widely, and the instructor makes choices about both based on the size of the group, the makeup of the group, and the needs of the group. An experienced teacher knows the type of presentation that is most effective in certain situations and uses this in planning the lesson.

The final step is to assess what the learner has learned and therefore the success of the teaching session. This may occur at the time of a teaching session or in follow-up sessions and may be by observation, questioning, or testing.

Online education is an increasingly popular method of presenting educational material, and it should be noted that the same process is followed when designing this type of instruction.[3]

Several observations that will assist the instructor in planning and conducting learning sessions are the following:

1. Learners hear and process information in individual ways. Repetition and variety in presentation means better reception.
2. Introduce key points early in the session and repeat as necessary.
3. The learners' previous knowledge influences what they learn in a new situation.
4. Present new information in small amounts at a time. Illustrate new concepts and facts with examples and easily understood terminology related to the workplace or class subject.
5. Encourage active learning by participation of the learner. Encourage questions, give time for discussion, and give assignments for future sessions or follow-up if applicable.

CAREER OPPORTUNITIES IN EDUCATION

While all dietitians do some teaching in whatever area of practice they are employed, there is a diversity of career areas in education that dietitians may pursue. These are discussed in the following sections.

Elementary and Secondary Schools

School-based nutrition education is incorporated into health and science classes in primary, middle, and high schools. A dietitian who teaches at these levels must meet state teacher training and certification requirements. Generally, those who teach grades K–12 have responsibilities that extend well beyond food, nutrition, and health.

Some state departments of education have nutrition education and training sections that often employ registered dietitians who have advanced degrees in education. Such positions include creating curricula to integrate nutrition with other subjects, developing teaching materials, identifying instructional resources, and training teachers to deliver nutrition education.

Job opportunities for dietitians in child nutrition programs affect dietitians from the lunchroom to the classroom. School-based health centers—rapidly growing models for the delivery of comprehensive primary health care in elementary, middle, and high schools—afford another opportunity for dietitians interested in working with children and adolescents.[4]

There is also a need in these school-based centers for dietitians certified by the CDR for weight management of children and adolescents.[5]

Colleges and Universities

There are teaching opportunities for dietitians in culinary institutes, technical schools, and 2- or 4-year colleges. Such positions are often associated with programs for chefs, food service supervisors, dietetic technicians, dietary managers, entry-level dietitians, and hospitality managers. The emphasis is on teaching in the classroom, laboratory, or practice setting. Course responsibilities may include food preparation and food science, basic and applied nutrition, meal management, cultural food practices, food service management and equipment, nutrition assessment and therapy, nutrition counseling and education, and community nutrition.

University faculty roles are quite varied. In addition to their teaching responsibilities, university faculty are required to conduct research and provide service within the institution, community, or profession. They advise students on academic choices and research, serve on committees, consult with community groups, share their expertise with the media and the public, and provide departmental and university leadership for nutrition-related initiatives.

Higher education can include teaching other groups of students. For example, some institutions offer nutrition courses for nondietetics majors to fulfill requirements for general education, teacher certification, or health and physical education. Programs in the allied health professions may include nutrition courses. Dietitians can teach courses in nutritional anthropology or epidemiology, often included as part of the master's degree in public health programs.

Medical and Dental Education

Some graduate-trained dietitians are engaged in medical and dental education. Such a role requires assertiveness and creativity to convince administrators of the unique contributions that dietitians have to offer in medical and dental education. For an emphasis on prevention and health promotion, nutrition is a required component, and dietitians are the best qualified persons to provide this education. An in-depth knowledge of nutrition science and medical nutrition therapy is required. Additionally, medical and dental nutrition educators must possess leadership ability, self-direction, strong communication skills, conceptual thinking skills, time management techniques, and flexibility.

Nutrition education can occur at any level of a medical or dental curriculum. It may consist of nutrition science with clinical application during the first 2 years while basic information is the major part of the curriculum. As students enter the clinical part of their program, sample meals featuring special diets are often effective teaching tools. Nutrition rounds and seminars can be incorporated when students are in residencies. Practicing dietitians can be involved in problem-based learning as an effective way to make nutrition relevant for future medical practice.

Nursing and Allied Health Nutrition Education

Nutrition services are often provided by nondietitians, depending on the practice setting and contributions of various health professionals. For example, nurses regularly monitor food intake, evaluate laboratory values indicative of nutritional status, and give patients nutritional advice. Dental hygienists and health educators often screen for health or nutritional problems and provide education and intervention. All health professionals should understand the role nutrition plays in wellness and disease prevention, and they need training on appropriate interventions. Nutrition is included in the curriculum for nurses' training programs, and dietitians often teach the courses.

Industry-Based Education

Companies that manufacture medical nutrition products often employ dietitians to provide technical and clinical information to the sales force and to other personnel, including clinicians, retail pharmacists, and educators of healthcare professionals. Dietitians may educate via telephone, webinars, written correspondence, electronic mail, and by personal visits. They may participate in developing video, audio, and slide programs; technical monographs; newsletters; brochures; and professional and patient education publications on topics of medical nutrition therapy.

Companies that manufacture institutional equipment, food products, supplemental products such as high-protein and other preparations for tube feedings, infant formula, and supplements for nutritional additives may also employ dietitians to help promote and demonstrate the use of the products.

Personal characteristics and skills necessary for success in industry-based education include technical and professional proficiency, ability to critically and objectively analyze issues, attention to detail, high work standards, skill in written and oral communications, adaptability, and ability to tolerate stress. Clearly, such positions require a proficiency in nutritional science, practitioner experience, conceptual and analytic skills, altruistic values, and a service ethic.

Work-Site Nutrition Education

As increased attention is given to the role of nutrition in health and disease prevention, more opportunities for dietitians will open in work-site wellness programs. These work sites may include manufacturing plants, insurance companies, and service organizations. Some of these positions will focus entirely on nutrition education and may include screening for nutritional risk, program development, leading classes and demonstrations, creating exhibits and displays, and evaluating the effectiveness of nutrition education initiatives. Dietitians in these positions may provide valuable experience for dietetic interns or other students as well.

Work-site education opportunities can also include coordinators of training in large dietetics departments or at the regional level of contract food and nutrition service companies. Dietitians in such roles may oversee a dietetic internship, coordinate in-service training for food service and other personnel, and direct training for students from affiliating programs. Individuals with the appropriate background may be promoted to director of training and development at the institutional or corporate level.

EDUCATOR ROLES

As shown in the CDR audit of dietetics practice, dietitians participate in many activities in which they teach employees, patients, allied health professionals, students, and consumers. A variety of approaches are used to reach the desired audience, all of which involve communication. Verbal interaction and nonverbal cues enter into the effectiveness of the message, and the skilled educator takes into account the best way to communicate with the learner. Several of the roles by which dietitians interact with learners are discussed in the following section.

Mentor

A mentor is a person who may teach verbally, by demonstration of particular activities or skills, role modeling, or a combination of these approaches. The mentoring relationship is a shared experience between a teacher and a learner. A mentor may be one's peer, an instructor, a trusted advisor, or anyone more skilled—think of the teenager who helps a parent or grandparent become computer literate. The mentor may also be described as a tutor in that one-on-one teaching is the method used.[6]

The Nutrition Entrepreneurs practice group conducts a mentorship program aimed toward matching volunteer mentors with other members who need guidance to make their vision a reality.[7] The mentor program offers rewards for both mentors and those mentored.

Coach

A coach is one who inspires and motivates others. Coaching is sometimes described as the role assumed with individuals who are already achieving at a high level and is simply positive feedback for continued high performance. The coaching role is effective when involvement and trust are created, expectations are clarified, performance is acknowledged, actions are challenged, and achievement is rewarded. The football coach is the classic example of one who performs all these functions in the expectation of having a winning team.

Coaching is similar to reflective teaching in that the teacher may demonstrate a new procedure or piece of information, and the learner repeats the procedure. The coach responds with advice, criticism, explanation, description, or further demonstration. The learner reflects and compares the new information to his or her previous knowledge and acts accordingly.

Preceptor

The preceptor is one who provides direction and instruction, supervised performance, and evaluation of the learners ability in applied practice. The dietitian who oversees a dietetic intern in supervised practice has the title of preceptor. A preceptor must have good interpersonal and time-management skills as well as subject-matter competence as a skilled practitioner. Preceptors are essential in dietetics education and to the future of dietetic practice. They should consult and follow the *Standards of Practice and Standards of Professional Performance for Registered Dietitians (Generalist, Specialty, Advanced) in Education of Dietetics Practitioners* developed by the American Dietetic Association and educators to guide their practice.[8]

Many benefits are realized by both the preceptor and the student as well as the department or institution providing experiences for the student. Among the benefits for preceptors observed in one study were assisting students with application of knowledge and expertise, gaining personal satisfaction, observing students' growth from novice to practitioner, and stimulating ongoing interest in the profession.[9] Students gained valuable knowledge from the example set by experienced professionals and were guided to levels of achievement that allowed them to assume entry-level positions well prepared. The preceptor role was investigated by Winham et al[10] regarding the attitudes and perceptions held by a large sample of registered dietitians. While the value of the preceptor role was highly perceived, several areas were identified as possible target activities that would further enhance the experience and encourage others to assume the role.

Descriptions of the various roles as perceived by the teacher, preceptor/ teacher, preceptor/mentor, and mentor are shown in **Table 13-2**.

Table 13-2.   Preceptor Roles

	Preceptor/ teacher	Preceptor	Preceptor/ mentor	Mentor
View of intern	View student as continued learner	View intern as a prospective coworker[b]		View intern as a colleague[b]
Conceptual focus	Focus on both theory and practice learning	Focus on practice-based learning[a]		
Prior knowledge	Assess intern's prior content knowledge[c]		Assume intern has necessary content knowledge[b]	
Theory/ practice	Combine basic subject matter with application	Demonstrate the incorporation of theory in practice[a]		Identify unwritten workplace policies and practices[b]
Learning experiences	Provide learning experiences of varied types	Suggest useful learning experiences to help intern achieve learning objectives[a]		Encourage intern to determine learning experiences to achieve objectives[c]

Table 13-2.   Preceptor Roles (Continued)

	Preceptor/ teacher	Preceptor	Preceptor/ mentor	Mentor
Ethical concerns	Discuss potential ethical issues[c]	Uses case studies to demonstrate	Identify actual ethical concerns[b]	
Strengths-weaknesses	Identify intern's strengths and weaknesses[a]		Help intern become aware of strengths and weaknesses[a]	
Progress evaluation	Evaluation of continued academic progress	Provide periodic feedback during internship		
Intern self-evaluation		Identify usefulness of self-evaluation[c]		Strongly encourage intern to participate in self-evaluation[c]
Role model	Illustrate role modeling by example	View yourself as a professional role model[a]		View yourself as a personal role model[a]
Duration of relationship	Recognize relationship with intern is limited[a]			View the relationship with the intern as indefinite[b]

Columns represent the categorical descriptions for each role. Rows represent the functions/ elements that relate to the supervised practice experience.

a. Practice preceptors indicated they "frequently" execute and do not want to change.

b. Practice preceptors executed in varying degrees from frequently or occasionally to seldom/ never, but do not want to change.

c. Practice preceptors believed they should do more often.

Data from *Journal of the American Dietetic Association* 102, Number 7 (July 2002), Wilson, M.A. "Dietetic Preceptors Perceive Their Role to Include a Variety of Elements," 969, Copyright 2002.

Counselor

Counseling is a process of listening, accepting, clarifying, and helping clients or students form conclusions and develop plans of action. The process is guided toward helping individuals learn about their needs and about methods of coping with them.

Motivational interviewing is defined as a way of helping others bring about behavior change, such as curbing addictive behaviors.[11] This technique was used in a study that led to increased fruit and vegetable intake by African Americans.[12] This type of counseling is also described as a directive, client-centered style for eliciting behavior change by helping clients explore and resolve ambivalence.

A cognitive interview technique is sometimes used to assist in understanding how audiences or individuals process information. Respondents are led through a survey or message and asked to respond with their thoughts, feelings, or ideas that come to mind. With this information, better messages are formed and valuation tools are targeted.[13]

Patient-centered counseling facilitates change by assessing patients' needs and tailoring the intervention to the patient's stage in the process of change, personal goals, and unique challenges.[14] Four steps are followed: assessment, advising, assisting, and follow-up. In step 1, the dietitian-counselor asks questions to determine present behaviors. Open-ended questions will help gain this information. (See **Table 13-3** for examples.) In step 2, advisement based on the assessment is given toward helping the person make changes. Assisting, in step 3, involves giving motivational statements and encouragement. Goals and specific skills such as self-monitoring and problem solving will also be discussed. In the final step, follow-up toward maintaining dietary change will be presented and attainment of earlier goals discussed. Further help will also be provided.

Communicator

Effective communication is of utmost importance in all areas of dietetics, and almost any job description will include the need to communicate at all levels in an organization with both groups and individuals. Professionals who develop verbal and written skills, along with listening skills, establish strong relationships with clients, patients, and staff.

Table 13-3. A Model for Open-Ended Questioning

Questions for assessing stage of change and motivation

How do you feel about your current diet?

What problems have you had because of your diet?

What would you like to change about your diet now?

Why would you like to change your diet now?

What concerns do you have about changing your diet now?

What reasons might you have to want to maintain your current diet?

Questions for assessing past experiences with dietary change

What changes have you made to your diet? How long did you maintain the changes? If so, for how long? If not, how long did you maintain the change?

How did you make changes in your diet? What helped?

What difficulties did you encounter? How did you handle them?

Questions about anticipated challenges or barriers to change

What could get in your way of attaining your goal?

What situations will make it hardest for you to achieve your goal?

What other situations might make it difficult for you to maintain your change?

Questions about strategies to cope with challenges or barriers to change

What could you do when you face this challenge?

What else could you do in the face of this challenge or barrier?

What could help you cope with this challenge? How?

What has been helpful in the past to deal with this barrier?

Who could help you cope with this challenge? How?

What has been helpful in the past to deal with this barrier?

Questions for goal setting

What are you willing to change in your diet now?

When? How often will you do this?

Where will you do it?

What will you have to do in advance to ensure that you are able to make and maintain this change?

How confident are you of your ability to make and maintain this change?

Questions for follow-up

How did you do with your plan?

What helped you stay on target?

What difficulties did you encounter?

Questions for assessing lapse and relapse

What made it difficult for you to stay with your plan?

How did you feel after that?

What else could you have done to stay on track?

What would you like to do now?

Reprinted from *Journal of the American Dietetic Association* 101, no. 3 (March 2001), Rosal, M.C., C.B. Ebbeling, I. Lofgren, J.K. Ockene, I.S. Ockene, and J.R. Hebert. "Facilitating Dietary Change: The Patient-Centered Counseling Model," 333, Copyright 2001, with permission from Elsevier.

There are, at a minimum, seven components of the communication process. The components are as follows:

1. *Source.* The source is the starting point for information exchange.
2. *Message.* The message is the idea or information transmitted verbally or nonverbally.
3. *Channel.* The channel is the pathway for messages between the sender and the receiver.
4. *Receiver.* The receiver takes in the message, assigns meaning, interprets, and responds to the message.
5. *Feedback.* Feedback refers to the response from the receiver to the sender.
6. *Environment.* The environment is the context in which the message occurs, such as physical surroundings and cultural, historic, or attitudinal factors.
7. *Noise.* Noise is any aural, visual, or internal factor that can distract from the meaning of the message.

The communication methods that ensure messages are received need to be carefully selected. Professionals who provide nutrition information to the public will choose methods such as television, Internet, or printed materials. The development of dietary guidance messages through the use of focus groups and surveys of consumers is described by Borra et al.[15] In the consumer message development model (**Figure 13-1**), the issues are defined, the message developed and assessed, then fine-tuned and validated.

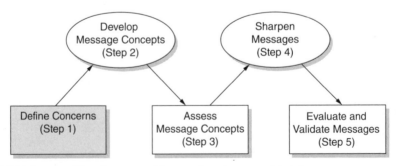

FIGURE 13-1. The Consumer Message Development Model.

Modified from Journal of the American Dietetic Association 101, Number 6 (June 20010, Borra, S., L. Kelly, M. Tuttle, and K. Neville. "Developing Actionable Dietary Guidance Messages: Dietary Fat as a Case Study," 679, Copyright 2001.

Today, while the use of e-mail, voice mail, and other social media are efficient, it should be emphasized that face-to-face communication is still important in many situations.[16] Human contact, especially in direct contact with patients, is the most reliable way of assuring the message is received because interaction can occur at the same time and reaction to the message assessed.

In a study to determine the best means of communicating nutrition education for elderly adults, several factors were found to be successful.[17] They included limiting educational messages to one or two, reinforcing and personalizing messages, providing purposeful activities and incentives, providing access to health professionals, and using behavior change. A model was developed showing these elements (**Figure 13-2**).

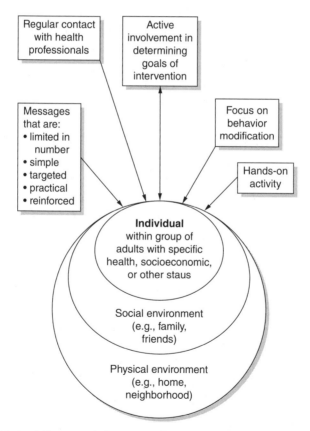

FIGURE 13-2. A Framework for a Nutrition Intervention.

Modified from Journal of the American Dietetic Association 104, Number 1 (January 2004), Sayhoun, N.R., C.A. Pratt, and A. Anderson. "Evaluation of Nutrition Education Interventions for Older Adults: A Proposed Framework," 66, Copyright 2004.

TYPES OF LEARNING

Education programs are based on learning outcomes or categories of learning, described as domains of learning. One classification, often used in education, describes five types of learning outcomes or skills as follows[18]:

1. *Psychomotor skills*. The learner acquires motor skills along with the know-how to perform tasks.
2. *Intellectual skills*. Information-processing skills allow the learner to perform a new activity.
3. *Verbal processing skills*. The learner is able to provide information through stating, listing, or describing something.
4. *Attitudinal skills*. The learner makes choices or decisions to act in certain ways. These may include long-term goals that determine a person's ability to perform psychomotor or other skills.
5. *Cognitive skills*. The learner has attained abstract strategies to become self-directed through the use of intellectual skills.

Another so-called index of learning styles[19] describes the following eight types of learning:

1. *Active*. An active learner likes trying things out and enjoys working in groups.
2. *Reflective*. A reflective learner thinks things through; he or she prefers working alone or with one or two partners.
3. *Sensing*. A sensing learner is concrete, practical, and oriented towards facts and procedures.
4. *Intuitive*. An intuitive learner is conceptual, innovative, and oriented toward theories and underling meanings.
5. *Visual*. A visual learner prefers visual representations or presented material.
6. *Verbal*. A verbal learner prefers written and spoken explanations.
7. *Sequential*. A sequential learner undertakes a linear thinking process and prefers learning in incremental steps.
8. *Global*. A global learner undertakes a holistic thinking process and prefers to learn in large steps.

Education through the use of methods that involve the learner in an active, participatory way can lead to very effective outcomes. Internships are examples of service learning. Problem-based learning is the method by which a student discovers new knowledge through individual learning in solving a problem. Project-based learning, similar to problem-based, is the method in which learner involvement is guided by an instructor. These three types of learning are described in the following sections.

Service Learning

Service learning is the type of educational experience that combines explicit academic learning with service.[20] In many professions, combining classroom study and community learning experiences is a way of enhancing and retaining learning. In dietetics, the internship is an example because it combines practice with instruction. Another example is the college class that places students in a community site such as a school or elderly nutrition program for experiences that are a part of the course requirements. Seeing and experiencing nutrition applied in specific community programs makes subject matter come alive and leads to a better understanding of the value and need of community service.

Problem-Based Learning

A method often used in medical and business schools, problem-based learning requires students to work through problems to find answers to real-life situations. This provides a context for students to learn critical thinking and problem-solving skills and to acquire knowledge of the essential concepts of a course of study.[21] In this method, students are presented a problem and organized into groups to discuss the problem. Students pose questions and rank the learning issues generated in the session. Students and the instructor discuss the resources needed to research the learning issues. Students then summarize their knowledge and connect the new concepts to older ones and define new learning issues as they progress through the problem. The benefit is that students recognize that learning is an ongoing process with new learning issues to be explored. Case-based learning is a method of problem-based learning designed to connect education and specialized practice while also developing skill for entry-level practice.[22]

The role of the instructor is to guide, probe, and support students' initiatives. When faculty incorporate problem-based learning into classes, they empower students to take a responsible role in their learning. As a result, faculty must be ready to yield some authority to their students.

Project-Based Learning

Similar to problem-based learning, project-based learning is a form of instruction that places emphasis on the students' involvement in working through job-related situations. It is described as a long-term, problem-focused, meaningful unit of instruction that integrates concepts from a number of disciplines. An example might be the design of a kitchen layout using work flow, equipment, and production schedules. Both teacher and student receive support in fulfilling their roles, the teacher as facilitator and shepherd of projects, and the student by participating in a worthwhile project. A project-based learning support system that supports learning through a computer-mediated interface using learner-centered software has been described.[23] This type of learning is useful in simulations or when students share a concentrated experience. New tools and structures are often needed to support the effectiveness of this type of learning, but it provides good results amid complex and challenging projects.

ADULTS AS LEARNERS

Conducting learning sessions for adults is different from teaching younger people. Dietitians need to be aware of the differences in order to adapt their teaching for the best learning outcomes. Adult learners, for example, have backgrounds of experience they bring to new learning situations and they are usually independent and self-directed. They may prefer to work alone or in small groups. Participating in activities and solving problems are typical preferences for learning styles as they may have immediate need for the information. Adults are often motivated by factors such as the need for an educational undertaking for economic or professional advancement reasons, a desire to learn new material, and for personal satisfaction. Even health reasons may factor into adult choices with the research showing that mental capacity is more readily maintained when the mind continues to be used throughout life.

TEACHING GROUPS AND TEAMS

Groups of people usually act in ways that are different than when they are in a one-on-one learning situation. *Group dynamics* is a term often applied to this behavior because it describes how members relate to each other, how they communicate among themselves, and how they work as a group. The teacher or leader of the group needs to understand how these dynamics can affect the learning process and the ways the educational message needs to be delivered.

Groups function best when all members participate because information is more likely to be shared and understood as new ideas, questions, clarifications, etc., occur. All group members need to understand the purpose and expected outcomes of the learning situation, and the leader has the responsibility to make sure this is clear at the outset of the lesson. When disagreements or tension arise in the group, the leader should be prepared to change the subject or take a time-out or use some other technique to get the group back on track. Giving support, encouraging discussion, and including all the group members in active participation helps ensure the session will accomplish its goals.

While teams are focused as a work group, many of the same characteristics as evidenced in groups will also appear. Teams may be formed in order to accomplish more through the combined efforts and expertise of individual members. Participation in teams, however, requires that members understand their role and the expectations for the group.

When teams are formed, members may be uncertain of their role and will depend on a leader to guide them into a team role. There may be conflict as team members clarify the team's goals. The leader then needs to redirect the energies of the team by encouraging open communication. As relationships become cohesive, the team functions as a unit and develops patterns of communication and behavior. The leader facilitates decision making and problem solving. The team members find ways of handling conflict, and methods that become standards for evaluating team performance therefore develop.

SUMMARY

The role of educator is one of the most important of those performed by the dietitian and dietetic technician. To be an effective educational leader, the professional must have a working knowledge of the education process by assessing learners' basic knowledge, setting learning goals, planning learning content and delivery methods, and evaluating the outcomes of the learning.

The dietitian may function in a number of educator roles, including that of mentor, coach, preceptor, or counselor. The effective teacher in any of these roles is skilled in communications and has the qualities of a leader in understanding individuals and groups and fostering productive learning situations.

DEFINITIONS

Assessment. The process of evaluating actions or conditions to base additional activity.

Cognitive skills. The application of intellectual capabilities to accomplish objectives.

Education. The systematic instruction and training designed to impart knowledge and develop a skill.

Instruction. The activity by which knowledge or teaching is imparted.

Psychomotor skills. The ability to perform physical tasks based on knowing or thinking.

Training. Actions by which persons are brought to a desired standard of efficiency or behavior by instruction and practice.

REFERENCES

1. Boyce, B. "2011 Future Connections Summit on Dietetic Practice, Credentialing, and Education: Summary of Presentations on Shaping the Future of the Dietetic Profession." *J Am Diet Assoc* 111 (2011): 1591–1599.
2. Ward, B., D. Rogers, C. Mueller, R. Touger-Decker, and K.L. Sauer. "Entry-Level Dietetics Practice Today: Results from the 2010 Commission of Dietetic Registration Entry-Level Dietetics Practice Audit." *J Am Diet Assoc* 111 (2011): 914–941.
3. Sandon, L. "A System for Designing Effective Online Education." *J Am Diet Assoc* 107 (2007): 1305–1306.
4. "Position of the American Dietetic Association, School Nutrition Association, and Society for Nutrition Education: Comprehensive School Nutrition Services." *J Am Diet Assoc* 110 (2010): 1738–1749.
5. American Dietetic Association. "Certificate of Training in Childhood and Adolescent Weight Management." Accessed December 1, 2015, www.eatright.org
6. Managan, L. "The Many Modes of Mentoring: New Spins on the Classic Relationship." *J Acad Nutr Diet* 112, no. 9 (2012): 1324–1328.
7. Bitzer, R., Nutrition Entrepreneurs Practice Group. "Mentor Program." *Ventures* XXV, no. 4 (2009): 11.
8. Anderson, J.A., K. Kennedy-Hagen, M.R. Stieber, D.S. Hollingsworth, K. Kattelman, C.L. Stein-Arnold, and B.M. Egan. "Dietetics Educators of Practitioners and Dietetic Association Standards of Professional Performance for Registered Dietitians (Generalist, Specialty/Advanced) in Education of Dietetics Practitioners." *J Am Diet Assoc* 109 (2009): 747–754.

9. Marincic, P.Z., and E.E. Francfort. "Supervised Program Preceptors' Perceptions of Rewards, Benefits, Support, and Commitment to the Preceptor Role." *J Am Diet Assoc* 102 (2002): 543–545.

10. Winham, D.M., A.A. Wooden, A.M. Hutchins, L.M. Morse, C.M. Shepard, S. Mayal-Kreiser, and J. Hempl. "Attitudes and Perception of the Dietetic Internship Preceptor Role by Arizona Nutrition Professionals." *Topics in Clinical Nutrition* 29, no. 3 (2014): 210–226.

11. Thorpe, M. "Motivational Interviewing and Dietary Behavior Change." *J Am Diet Assoc* 103 (2003): 150–151.

12. Resicow, K., A. Jackson, T. Wang, F. McCarty, W.W. Dudley, and T. Baranowski. "A Motivational Interviewing Intervention to Increase Fruit and Vegetable Intake Through Black Churches; Results of the Eat for Life Trial." *Am J Public Health* 91 (2001): 1686–1693.

13. Carbone, E.T., M.K. Campbell, and L. Honess-Morreal. "Use of Cognitive Interview Techniques in the Development of Nutrition Surveys and Interactive Messages for Low-Income Populations." *J Am Diet Assoc* 102 (2002): 690–696.

14. Rosal, M.C., C.B. Ebbeling, I. Lofgren, J.K. Ockene, I.S. Ockene, and J.R. Hebert. "Facilitating Dietary Change: The Patient-Centered Counseling Model." *J Am Diet Assoc* 101 (2001): 332–341.

15. Borra, S., L. Kelly, M. Tuttle, and K. Neville. "Developing Actionable Dietary Guidance Messages: Dietary Fat as a Case Study." *J Am Diet Assoc* 101 (2001): 678–684.

16. Hallowell, E.M. "The Human Moment at Work." *Harvard Bus Review* (January–February 1999): 1–8.

17. Sayhoun, N.R., C.A. Oratt, and A. Anderson. "Evaluation of Nutrition Education Interventions for Older Adults: A Proposed Framework." *J Am Diet Assoc* 101 (2001): 58–69.

18. Gagne, R.M. *Instructional Technology: Foundations.* (Hillsdale, NJ: Lawrence Erlbaum Associates, 1987): 25.

19. Palermo, C., K.Z. Walker, T. Brown, and M. Zogi. "How Dietetics Students Like to Learn: Implications for Curriculum Planners." Dietitians Association of Australia. *J Compilation* (2009).

20. Kim, Y., and A. Canfield. "How to Develop a Service Learning Program in Dietetics Education." *J Am Diet Assoc* 102 (2002): 174–176.

21. Dietetic Educators of Practitioners Practice Group. "Problem-Based Learning: Preparing Students to Succeed in the 21st Century." *DEP Line* 17, no. 3 (1998): 1–5.

22. Harman, T., B. Bertrand, A. Green, A. Pettus, J. Jennings, E. Wall-Bassett, and O.T. Babatunde. "Case-Based Learning Facilitates Critical Thinking in Undergraduate Nutrition Education: Students Describe the Big Picture." *J Acad Nutr Diet* 115, no. 3 (2015): 378–388.

23. Laffey, J., T. Tupper, D. Musser, and J. Wedman. "A Computer-Mediated Support for Project-Based Learning." *Technology Research and Development* 46, no. 1 (1998): 73–86.

CHAPTER 14

The Dietitian as Researcher

"Research is the foundation of our profession."[1]

OUTLINE

LEARNING OBJECTIVES

The student will be able to:
1. Gain information about research goals of the Academy.
2. Understand the importance of research in dietetics.
3. Become familiar with the ways dietitians can participate in research in all areas of practice.
4. Know practical applications of evidence-based and outcome research.

INTRODUCTION

Many dietitians conduct research as a part of their work. This is especially true for dietitians who specialize in nutrition support, pediatrics, renal dietetics, oncology, AIDS, or diabetes. These dietitians and those in all other areas of practice use research in various ways. They may critique and use research data for professional reference as needed. All dietitians are encouraged to perform or collect data for outcome research studies to demonstrate the effectiveness of medical nutrition therapy and/or the quality and acceptance of the services performed. In the clinical setting, dietitians may collaborate with physicians who are conducting nutrition-related studies, and even though they may not call themselves researchers, they are in fact participating in research and are critical to the process.

With the increasing emphasis on research in the Academy of Nutrition and Dietetics and in the profession generally, many dietitians are incorporating research studies into their practice. In part, there is a sense that more applied research studies are needed as more basic, laboratory-oriented research does not always meet the needs of everyday practice. To this end, a member network called the Dietetics Practice-Based Research Network (DPBRN) has been formed.[2] The network is open to all who are interested in addressing questions encountered in practice and to continually improve the delivery of food and nutrition services.

IMPORTANCE OF RESEARCH IN DIETETICS

"Research represents the future for dietetics; it is the foundation for our credibility, our recognition, and our professional respect. Without research, we cannot properly educate or advocate, nor would we have the credibility in either endeavor."[3] All professions continually reshape themselves to meet ever-changing needs in society and research is essential for these changes and advancements to take place. Not only do dietitians need to engage in research to gain knowledge and define new modes of therapy and new techniques in all areas of practice, they also need to take a scholarly approach to everyday practice. Many practicing dietitians have an image of research as overwhelming or irrelevant, when in fact the reality is quite different. There are a number of exciting ways for practicing dietitians to become involved with research, ranging from simply learning more about dietetics-related research, to evaluating research findings to make evidence-based decisions in work settings and participating in scientific projects.[4]

Employers of dietitians and those using dietetic services need to be assured that the services they are using are supported by research. Research is the basis for education because it drives the core knowledge and competencies and is used in setting public policy. The ability to conduct and use research further allows professionals to be recognized by the public as a valued and credible source of scientifically supported nutrition information.

The Academy has taken further steps to encourage and increase research by creating a software platform to advance evidence-based research called the Academy of Nutrition and Dietetics Health Informatics infrastructure (ANDHII); the program provides for a collection of data about dietetic practice on a national scale and makes it available for outcomes research and quality improvement.[5]

THE RESEARCH PHILOSOPHY OF THE ACADEMY

The research philosophy of the profession is the following:

> The Academy of Nutrition and Dietetics believes that research is the foundation of the profession, providing the basis for practice, education, and policy. Dietetics is the integration and application of principles derived from the sciences of nutrition, biochemistry, physiology, food management, and behavioral and social sciences to achieve and

maintain people's health; therefore dietetics research is a dynamic collaborative and assimilative endeavor. This research is broad in scope, ranging from basic to applied practice research.[6]

The Academy uses research as the basis of decisions, policy, and communication in a variety of roles. The roles include the following:

- *Advocate.* Federal and nongovernmental agencies, organizations, and individuals who can support the Academy's research agenda.
- *Facilitator.* Targets key research questions and facilitates a successful process to answer the questions.
- *Convener.* Brings together scientists and practitioners from various disciplines to explore new approaches in solving research questions.
- *Funder.* Prepares, disseminates, and funds research proposals on key research questions important to the profession.
- *Educator.* Develops professional opportunities for members to enhance their knowledge and use of research.
- *Disseminator.* Distributes research results to members and the public through publications, work sites, and print and electronic media.

THE ACADEMY'S RESEARCH PRIORITIES

The Research Committee

The Research Committee of the Academy, reporting to the board of directors and the house of delegates (HOD), sets the research agenda for the Academy. In this capacity, the committee develops, maintains, and evaluates the research priorities.[7] The Academy's statement of purpose emphasizes research: "The Academy is committed to improving the nation's health and advancing the profession of dietetics through research, education, and advocacy."[8] Two specific strategies to help reach these goals are to equip members to use research in their work and provide research and resources that can be translated into evidence-based practice.

In 2014, the research committee identified priority research areas as the following:

- Prevention and treatment of obesity and chronic diseases.
- Nutrition and lifestyle education.
- Nutritional status and disease risk assessment.
- Translational nutrition.

- Nutrition and genetics.
- Provision of dietetic services.
- Customer satisfaction.
- Education and retention of dietetic practitioners.
- Safe, secure, and sustainable food supply.

Funding for approved projects comes from the Academy foundation and other Academy-affiliated groups, from governmental agencies, and from the food and nutrition industry. A tool kit that provides a lesson tutorial, practice suggestions, and resources for conducting research is available from the headquarters office.

Figure 14-1 illustrates the interaction between practice, education, and policy.

Research Dietetic Practice Group

The Research Dietetic practice group has over 650 members from a variety of work settings, including clinical research centers, nonprofit groups, governmental agencies, universities, and many practice areas. Membership is open to all Academy members who conduct research or are interested in research. Members collaborate on Academy projects, such as the Evidence Analysis Library, to bring together research from many sources, and in the preparation of position papers.

Members of this group also form liaisons with the Research Committee of the Association and the DPBRN. The practice group provides a member network, conducts continuing professional education events, provides a packet of information for new members, and produces a website and a periodic publication. Research awards are given to recognize the research and publications generated by members.

Dietetics Practice-Based Research Network

The Dietetics Practice-Based Research Network (DPBRN) brings practitioners and researchers together to identify research that is needed in practice settings, design significant research to obtain funding, and carry research into real-life practice. The focus of the research conducted by members is in studies that can be immediately incorporated into practice. Professionals who lack the time, money, or perhaps experience to conduct research on their own find that this group activity presents an opportunity to benefit from research by answering questions, keeping abreast of new information, and improving their practice.

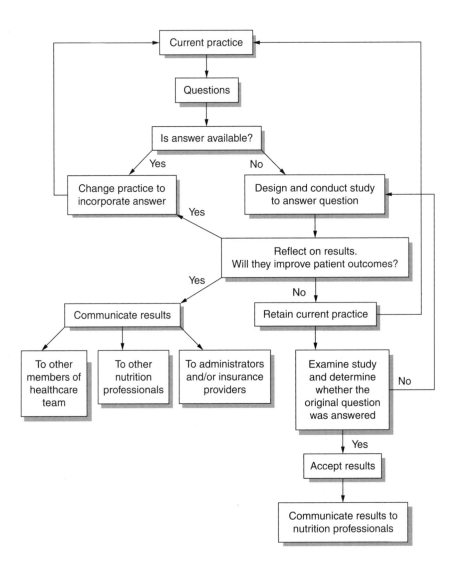

FIGURE 14-1. Detailed Progression of How Research and Clinical Practice are Integrated.

Reprinted from *Journal if the American Dietetic Association* 89, Number 4, 1998. Eck LH, Slawson DO, Williams R, Smith K, Harmon-Clayton K, Oliver D, "A Model for Making Outcomes Research Standard Practice in Clinical Dietetics. Copyright 1998, with permission from Elsevier.

RESEARCH APPLICATIONS

Evidence-Based Practice

Evidence-based practice, based on evidence-based research, is the integration of the best available evidence from reviewed research with professional expertise and client values to make food and nutrition practice decisions.[8] Every area of practice in dietetics involves making decisions about the best procedures to follow, and given that new information continually leads to a need to make necessary changes or to update practice, evidence analysis provides this information. The evidence analysis process involves the following steps:

1. Formulate one or more questions to be researched.
2. Conduct a literature search for each question.
3. Critically appraise each report found in the literature as to the quality of the research and the findings.
4. Summarize the evidence.
5. Develop conclusions and assign a grade based on the strength of the evidence.
6. Put into practice.

The Evidence Analysis Library at the Academy headquarters is maintained for the benefit of members of the Academy and others needing the information. The best and most relevant nutrition information is reviewed and is available in this accessible, user-friendly library.[9] Because of the research data held, governmental and other groups also use the information and the process in making policy decisions. One example group is the Food and Drug Administration, which uses the process to make decisions about the use of health claims on food labels.

Outcomes research is increasingly important in the linkage of practice and research in order to make advancements in all areas of dietetics. Currently, translational research is being used in much the same way as outcomes research, that is, to link research to practice applications in all areas. Van Horn points out the value of clinical nutrition outcomes research and the involvement of dietitians in a letter in the journal.[10] Surveys show that while dietitians consider research important and are interested in it, many experience obstacles to performing outcomes research because of a lack of knowledge about the process, along with limited time and funding.[11,12]

Dietetic educators and university faculty have also experienced barriers to research activities even though research is required of most faculty.[13]

INVOLVEMENT IN RESEARCH

The Commission on Dietetic Registration conducts periodic audits of practice areas of RDs and DTRs. Data was collected for entry-level practitioners and is shown in **Table 14-1**. While the 2015 Compensation and Benefits Survey indicated that only 6 percent of RDs and 2 percent of DTRs are employed in education and research, the higher involvement in specific research-related activities in the practice audit would be expected to represent activities performed as a part of the job but not as the major area of employment.[14] The fact that dietetic technicians also participate in some research activities very likely reflects degrees obtained beyond the basic technician education requirements as well as job responsibilities.

CAREER OPPORTUNITIES IN RESEARCH

Many university-affiliated hospitals have centers dedicated to types of clinical research. Others have long-term, multidisciplinary research projects that include a nutrition component. Some dietitians work at a general clinical research center (GCRC), usually associated with an academic medical center and federally funded. There are about 80 GCRCs funded by the National Institutes of Health located at universities across the country.

Research dietitians may oversee the metabolic kitchens associated with the GCRCs, analyze nutrient intakes, conduct calorimetry studies, assist in the development of nutrition-related protocols, and participate in rounds and seminars.

Some GCRC dietitians manage their own research programs, direct nutrition research, and collaborate with the medical school faculty in research. Some large national studies provide numerous opportunities for dietitians to become involved as nutrition counselors, data managers, or project directors.

There is a need for dietitians in clinical research. The best dietetics practice must be based on scientific principles and sound theory. Recent activities of the National Institutes of Health support these concepts.[15] In an attempt to advance the translation research activities into new drugs, equipment, new therapies for diseases, and prevention, it has established

Table 14-1. Research Activities of RDs and DTRs

	Percent involved in any way	
	RD	DTR
Evaluate and synthesize research literature	19	10
Use evidence analysis in practical decisions	76	32
Review research literature	54	21
Evaluate and synthesize research literature	19	10
Use evidence analysis in practice decisions	76	32
Review research literature	54	21
Collect data for research	24	0
Analyze data	42	0
Write grant proposals	36	0
Develop hypotheses for research studies	5	0
Design research studies	6	0
Develop research proposals	5	0
Conduct research studies	8	0
Report research at professional conferences	6	0
Write manuscripts for peer-reviewed journals	5	0
Review and use national nutrition survey data	29	0
Identify nutrition-related problems within population groups	12	0
Collect data for research	24	0
Analyze data	42	0
Write grant proposals	36·	0
Develop hypotheses for research studies	5	0
Design research studies	6	0
Develop research proposals	5	0
Conduct research studies	8	0

Reprinted from *Journal of the American Dietetic Association* 111, no. 11 (November 2011), Ward, B., D. Rogers, C. Mueller, R. Touger-Decker, KI.L. Sauer, C. Schmidt, "Distinguishing Entry-Level RD and DTR Practice: Results from the 2010 Commission on Dietetic Registration Entry-Level Dietetics Practice Audit, 1749–1755, Copyright 2011, with permission from Elsevier.

the National Center for Advancing Translational Science (NCATS). This center will fund projects and translational science centers all over the nation, which will provide dietitians and nutrition scientists with opportunities to collaborate with other scientists and compete for grants in applied research as basic science. Additional evidence is needed to support the value of many approaches to clinical dietetics. Additional knowledge is needed in areas of nutritional status of individuals and populations at risk for disease, genetic components of disease related to food intake patterns, identification of nutrient requirements associated with disease conditions, environmental risks (including dietary risks), nutrition interventions as therapy for disease conditions, and eating behavioral research. With the crises in healthcare delivery, especially in adult and childhood obesity, the outcomes of nutrition intervention are an important area of investigation.

Food and Industry Companies

Many food companies employ dietitians. Roles vary but include research related to product or recipe development. Roles can also focus on translation of research into meaningful information for the public or development of nutrition education for children, adults, and professionals.

Companies that manufacture infant formulas and medical nutritional products often employ dietitians to conduct research or to monitor clinical investigations in hospitals, nursing homes, and home care settings. Roles might include work related to:

- Nutritional needs of infants, children, and the elderly
- Acceptability of flavors and textures of products designed for oral use
- Coordination of studies to determine the effectiveness of new products
- Initiation of outcomes research to explore the cost-effectiveness of medical nutrition therapy

Government

There are many opportunities for research dietitians in government-sponsored centers and laboratories. These include positions such as:

- Nutrition scientists at the Department of Agriculture laboratories studying nutrient requirements, vitamins and minerals, eating pattern interventions, and other nutrition topics

- Researchers at the U.S. Army Natick Research, Development, and Engineering Center in Massachusetts involved in studies related to food behaviors and the acceptance and consumption of military rations
- Nutrition epidemiologists at the Centers for Disease Control and Prevention in Atlanta, Georgia, exploring patterns of nutrition-related-diseases and nutrition surveillance throughout the country
- Life science specialists at the Congressional Research Service in the Library of Congress, answering questions and conducting research for members of Congress and staff on food and nutrition issues
- Nutrition researchers at the National Aeronautical and Space Administration in Houston studying nutrition needs of space explorers

Community and Public Health

Since the leading causes of death in the United States continue to be nutrition-related chronic diseases, more efforts and opportunities are rising in community and population-based nutrition research. As consumers become more aware of disease consequences of their food choices and eating behaviors, they demand more evidence. Many dietitians who previously worked only in service program areas in community and public health are seizing the opportunity for research activities that document the value of nutrition and the dietitians' role in interventions. Great opportunities exist in conjunction with the obesity epidemic in getting individuals and communities involved in the food environment and in interventions that really change eating behaviors and adherence to dietary recommendations.

Schools are involved in research especially suited for nutrition, healthy behaviors, and weight maintenance by providing researchers access to students that they can follow over time. Dietitians will be needed in greater numbers for these research and education programs to be successful.

Many land-grant universities are conducting nutrition research in developing countries around the world. This research involves food and agriculture production, economic development, and nutritional assessment and intervention in various populations. As more and more globalization occurs, these ventures will increase, thus providing even greater opportunities for dietitians in research.

Human Nutrition Research Centers

The Agricultural Research Service of the U.S. Department of Agriculture funds six human nutrition research centers. These include the Children's Nutrition Research Center at Baylor College of Medicine in Houston, Texas, and the Arkansas Children's Nutrition Center at Arkansas Children's Hospital at the University of Arkansas for Medical Sciences. The center in Boston, Massachusetts, specializes in nutrition research for the aging population and is associated with Tufts University. Located on the campus of the University of California at Davis, the Western Human Nutrition Research Center concentrates on nutrition intervention strategies. The center in Beltsville, Maryland, conducts basic and applied research on nutrient composition, national dietary surveys, nutrient requirements, function of physiochemicals, and similar studies. The sixth center, located in Grand Forks, North Dakota, is associated with the University of North Dakota and conducts research in mineral requirements and utilization as well as community-based research with Native Americans. Opportunities are available at these centers for all levels of dietetic practice (entry level, advanced, specialists, and dietetic technicians) and include clinical trials, basic science and applied research, and community-based research.

INFORMATION SOURCES

An excellent source for information about types of research and research methodology with an emphasis in nutrition is *Research: Successful Approaches* by Monsen and Van Horn.[16] The *Journal of the Academy of Nutrition and Dietetics* provides valuable research articles and opportunities identifying other dietetic researchers along with opportunities to publish. Other useful sources for dietitians conducting or planning research feature qualitative research,[17] publishing research,[18–20] and scientific integrity.[21,22] The Research Dietetics practice group offers opportunities for collaboration, networking, and mentoring for various kinds of research.

SUMMARY

Researchers may be based in specialized clinical research centers, government agencies, industry, universities, or the workplace. Roles vary according to the employing institution's mission and purpose. Key areas of investigation relate to nutrient requirements, nutrient utilization, and outcomes of medical nutrition therapy. Opportunities for participating in outcomes research in order to enhance practice exist through collaborative research that utilizes the expertise of dietitians in many practice settings. All dietitians can benefit from research findings applied to practice and can utilize the Academy's Evidence Analysis Library for the current and best research.

DEFINITIONS

Evidence-based research. The compilation of research studies that, together, allows for a decision regarding application to practice.

Outcomes research. Studies that focus on results of interventions and application of research results.

Research. Systematic investigation leading to new knowledge or new applications of known information. To conduct research, a question is formulated, a literature search is conducted, experimental activities are applied, and results are recorded.

REFERENCES

1. Pavlinac, J.M. "President's Page." *J Am Diet Assoc* 110 (2010): 499.
2. Trostler, N., E.F. Meyer., and L.N. Snetselaar. "Description of Practice Characteristics and Professional Activities of Dietetics Practice-Based Research Network Members." *J Am Diet Assoc* 108 (2008): 1060–1067.
3. Yadrick, M. "President's Page." *J Am Diet Assoc* 108 (2008): 11601.
4. See Note 1.
5. Murphy, W.J. "New Breed of Evidence and the Tools to Generate It: Introducing ANDHII" *J Acad Nutr Diet* 115, no. 1 (2015): 19–22.
6. www.eatright.org (1/9/16).
7. See Note 5.
8. Vaughn, L.A., and C.J.J. Manning. "Meeting the Challenges of Dietetics Practice with Evidence-Based Decisions." *J Am Diet Assoc* 104 (2004): 282–284.
9. Academy of Dietetics and Nutrition. "Evidence-Based Library." www.eatright.org
10. Van Horn, L. "Clinical Nutrition Research: New Approaches and New Outcomes." *Acad Nutr Diet J* (2012): 971.
11. McCaffree, J. "Overcoming Obstacles to Outcomes Research." *J Am Diet Assoc* 102 (2002): 71.
12. Hayes, J.E., and C.A. Peterson. "Use of an Outcomes Research Collaborative Training Curriculum to Enhance Entry-Level Dietitians and Established Professionals' Self-Reported Understanding of Research." *J Am Diet Assoc* 103 (2003): 77–81.

13. Whelan, K., and S. Markless. "Factors That Influence Research Involvement among Registered Dietitians Working as University Faculty: A Qualitative Interview Study." *J Acad Nutr Diet* 102 (2012): 1021–1028.
14. Rogers, D. "Compensation and Benefits Survey 2015." *J Acad Nutr Diet* 115, no. 3 (2015): 370–388.
15. U.S. Department of Health and Human Services. "NIH Establishes National Center for Advancing Translational Sciences." *NIH News*, press release, December 23, 2011.
16. Monsen, E.R., and L. Van Horn. *Research, Successful Approaches*, 3rd ed. (Chicago: American Dietetic Association, 2007).
17. Harris, J.E., G.P.M. Gleason, C. Boushey, J.A. Beto, and B. Bruemer. "An Introduction to Qualitative Research for Food and Nutrition Professionals." *J Am Diet Assoc* 109 (2009): 80–90.
18. Boushey, C., J. Harris, B. Bruemmer, S.A. Archer, and L. Van Horn. "Publishing Nutrition Research: A Review of Study Design, Statistical Analyses, and Other Key Elements of Manuscript Preparation. Part 1." *J Am Diet Assoc* 106 (2006): 89–96.
19. Harris, J.E., C.J. Boushey, B. Bruemmer, and S.A. Archer. "Publishing Nutrition Research: A Review of Nonparametric Methods." *J Am Diet Assoc* 108 (2008): 1488–1496.
20. Boushey, C.J., J. Harris, B. Bruemmer, and S.A. Archer. "Publishing Nutrition Research: A Review of Sampling, Sample Size, Statistical Analyses, and Other Key Elements of Manuscript Preparation. Part 2." *J Am Diet Assoc* 108 (2008): 679–688.
21. The International Life Sciences Institute North America Conflict of Interest/ Scientific Integrity Guiding Principles Working Group. "Funding Food Science and Nutrition Research: Financial Conflicts and Scientific Integrity." *J Am Diet Assoc* 109 (2009): 929–936.
22. Nicklas, T.S., W. Karmally, and C.E. O'Neil. "Nutrition Professionals Are Obligated to Follow Ethical Guidelines When Conducting Industry-Funded Research." *J Am Diet Assoc* 111 (2011): 1931–1932.

The Future in Dietetics and Nutrition

"This is the time for the science of nutrition.
This is the moment, and we have to seize it."
Bernadine Healy[1]

OUTLINE

LEARNING OBJECTIVES

1. Project future roles anticipated in the health care, the foods industry, nutrition research, private practice, and community nutrition.
2. Understand the range of future opportunities through changing technologies.
3. Discuss future educational needs as indicated by employers of dietitians.
4. Become familiar with the role of management and leadership in food service systems and other dietetic areas.
5. Understand the importance of informatics in dietetic practice.

INTRODUCTION

All organizations, of necessity, plan for the future in terms of goals, timelines, personnel, economic considerations, and the business/professional climate. The Academy of Nutrition and Dietetics (AND) expends a great deal of time and effort in all these areas. The House of Delegates, Accreditation Council on Education in Nutrition and Dietetics (ACEND), the Commission on Dietetic Registration (CDR), and the Foundation and the Board of Directors all participate in activities designed to identify and prepare for the future of the Academy and its members.

The House of Delegates has established a *mega issues process* as a "strategic and futuristic projection to impact the profession 3 to 5 years into the future." The Council on Future Practice works with both ACEND and CDR to anticipate and identify actions and needs for the future. In the Council's Visioning Report,[2] education, credentialing, and practice needs of the profession are outlined, with recommendations the Academy may take toward implementing the goals in these areas. The AND Foundation projects needs for funding scholarships and research for the Academy and works closely with business/industry groups for funding. The Board of Directors periodically appoints committees to investigate issues and conduct long-range planning seminars and workshops for leaders and members. Most recently, the AND Foundation was charged with developing a 100th anniversary strategy to celebrate the anniversary of the Academy. In 2014, a 100th Anniversary Steering Committee was identified to begin the planning and implementation strategies. Three issues were initially identified: RDNs (registered dietitian nutritionists) as global leaders in food systems; increased global capacity of nutrition professionals; and nutrition recognized as a central pillar of individual and public health.[3] These themes clearly represent the thinking of moving the Academy into the next 100 years and will impact future careers, practice, and education for dietetic practitioners.

As a part of the system-wide health field, the dietetics/nutrition profession is bound by the same practice needs identified by the Institute of Medicine as core competencies.[4] These are: patient-centered care, work in interdisciplinary teams, provision of evidence-based practice, application of quality improvement, and use of informatics.

In this chapter, issues important to the future of the Academy are emphasized. The general topics are: 1. Education, 2. Practice, 3. Communications and Technology, 4. Foods and the food supply, and 5. Management and productivity.

EDUCATION

Change is constant in response to dietetic practice needs. Numerous committees, study groups, surveys, and reports over the years attest to the intent to assure qualified practitioners now and in the future. Changes in health care, in food service, in community programs, and in governmental programs and policies have all impacted the profession, making it necessary to constantly examine the educational preparation of dietitian/nutritionists in all of these areas.

The Academy's Environmental Scan in 2012 identified in the Visioning Report, a need for more knowledge in emerging areas in nutrition and dietetics are identified as nutritional genomics, telehealth, nutritional pharmacology, case management, behavioral counseling, prescriptive authority, coding and reimbursement, evidence-based practice, and informatics. Also indicated in the Visioning Report, most health professions are now requiring the advanced degree and experience for entry-level practice. This will become a requirement in dietetics education in 2024 due to the advancement in the profession.[5]

There is a further need for all professionals to be educated to work more interprofessionally (partnering with other RDNs with unique skills and expertise), collaborate and network with other professional disciplines, apply evidence-based research, and business skills.[6]

The importance of interprofessional education is evidenced when there is coordination among all groups providing client services or health care. The Institute of Medicine has recommended an overhaul of the healthcare system, stating that all professionals should be educated to deliver patient-centered care as members of an interdisciplinary team.[7] This is true in most areas of future dietetic practice. For example, a rapidly growing area of senior retirement communities and independent living facilities will provide opportunities for RDNs and dietetics technician, registered (DTRs). The teams will be composed of RDNs, chefs, physical therapists, fitness trainers, occupational and speech therapists, and physicians as these communities seek to provide a complete continuum of care for the rapidly expanding number of "baby boomers" who choose a different lifestyle. These communities are more in tune with social models (lifestyle, health, wellness, physical activities, etc.) than the medical/clinical models of the past (nursing homes, etc.). Although RDNs have not moved quickly into these areas, their skill and knowledge are much needed in an atmosphere where the dining experience becomes the most important event of the day for many and it will not be served in apartments or at bedsides. In addition food and nutrition information is eagerly sought by the residents, particularly in regard to physical activity and staying active. Corporate management firms are forming to deliver these services and dietitians of the future must be involved.

Several universities now incorporate interprofessional experiences in education programs and cite a number of benefits that accrue as a result. Part-time work experiences, summer internships, travel abroad programs, student exchange programs, and shadowing of working professionals are examples of such experiences that give students valuable insights into the work world and future careers.

Educators are offering more degree options and emphases at all levels of study. As an example of what one university offers to expand student career options, the following are available:[8]

Degree Options

    i. Dietetics

    ii. Allied Health

    iii. Human Nutrition and Pre-medicine

    iv. Community Nutrition with Emphases in Nutrition and Exercise; Nutrition Education; School Nutrition and Exercise; Nutrition Education; School Nutrition and Food Service Management; Food, Nutrition and the Public

Emerging trends also point to the need for practitioners to continually acquire the necessary knowledge and skills throughout their working lives by continuing education through advanced degrees, workshops, seminars, webinars, distance program, and others.

PRACTICE

Societal trends, health care, public health policies, advances in communications, technology, and the biosciences all impact the practice of dietetics now and into the future.[9] As new and existing competitors become more aggressive in seeking to provide food and nutrition programs and seminars, RDNs must become more assertive with owning the food and nutrition profession. Trends such as these point to the need to be proactive in preparing for changing roles through educational and experiential means. Health educators and pharmacists continue to provide more food/nutrition information which is a perfect example of the need for RDNs to take leadership in these roles and pursue partnering and collaborating with these professionals as well as others.

RDNs must be able to recognize the need for their expertise in new areas and willing to try new career scenarios. These may include emergency feeding of immigrants or displaced groups; serving on health policy groups at all levels of government; collaborating with genetic and epidemiology researchers to ensure that the impact of food eaten and food composition is considered; assisting in rural health centers with assessment, treatment, and education of clients and professionals; working with foundations/agencies that fund community programs; and assisting in the development of small businesses relating to food and nutrition in rural areas. Another area not to be overlooked is the inclusion of the RDN in research in food and related community nutrition. An emerging role for RDNs is in promoting community organizations to involve and assist community citizens in the planning, implementing, and evaluating programs and research planned in their communities to achieve healthy communities.

As a result of the 2014, Centers of Medicare and Medicaid Services ruling, RDNs may write diet orders for modified diets and medical nutrition therapy including vitamin and mineral supplementation, enteral and parenteral nutrition, and can order nutritional laboratory tests.[10] The complex knowledge of pharmacology is needed to carefully select and time medical nutrition therapy in patients also receiving medication therapy.

It has been estimated that by the year 2050, 33 percent of the U.S. population will have diabetes mellitus.[11] Due to this predicted increase and changing healthcare models, RDNs will be increasingly called upon to provide services as a level 3 educator (uncertified educator of Diabetes Self-Management Education Provider—four levels) and DTRs will serve as level 2 educators. The emergence of nontraditional settings will require nutrition and dietetics positions to work in community health centers, faith-based institutions, public libraries, retail pharmacy clinics, congregate housing for the elderly, nephrology clinics, bariatric surgery practices, patient-centered medical homes, nurse-managed health centers, community nursing centers, telehealth, worksites, schools, and diabetes-related companies.

The U.S. Bureau of Labor Statistics has projected growth in demand for diabetes educators due to an expansion of federally qualified health centers and other community health centers from the Patient Protection and Affordable Care Act. Little work has been done at present on state licensure of diabetes educators and they are classified as "health educators" as there is no standard job classification by the U.S. government.[12]

Non-RD Practice

The Academy is faced with the reality that a large number of food and nutrition graduates do not become registered. This may be due to any of several reasons: lack of an internship appointment, geographical location, or for economic reasons. Colleges and universities share a responsibility with the association to advise students about the realities of the job market with and without the credential. Throughout several of the chapters in this book, suggestions are given for potential practice areas not requiring registration. The Academy has taken some steps to assist the non-RD, but this is a situation needing further focus and attention.

In 2013, Practice Audit of the Non-RD and DTR graduate,[13] 880 individuals indicated job titles currently held and activities performed. The survey gives insight into the types of positions held in clinical nutrition practice, in community nutrition, and in food and nutrition management. Only a few indicated a practice area in education and research or in consultation and business. As the career and client base continues to increase, RDNs will be in greater demand and will need to collaborate and partner with the DTRs and other noncertified food and nutrition graduates in order to meet the growing needs. For RDNs this means assuming leadership and moving into the "expert" roles, and delegating "novice," or beginning tasks to DTRs and others in order to maintain their position as the food/nutrition experts.

As the public of all ages (especially the large numbers of baby boomers) plus related professionals (MD, OT, PharmD, chefs, food companies, etc.) become more aware of the importance of nutrition and foods in health, wellness, disease prevention, activity levels, and even mental health, professional roles begin to blur. Again this is an indication that RDNs must be aggressive in presenting their skills and knowledge unique to this area.

Practice Needs

The focus of practice in all areas of food and nutrition is customer/client needs and preferences. It can be generally said that consumers are concerned about convenience, quality, personalization, cost, and accessibility. Leadership and business skills are highly valued in the profession as are innovation and entrepreneurship. As new practice opportunities arise that lead to new career choices, nutrition, and dietetics practitioners will need to be even more strategic in planning their educational pathways and careers.

There is a need for intensive, behavioral dietary counseling for persons with a range of risk factors for chronic diseases, especially cardiovascular disease as the major cause of death in the United States that can be delivered by nutrition and dietetics practitioners. Behavioral counseling, in turn, suggests a need for increased skill in counseling, motivational interviewing, coordination of care, and program planning.[14] Medical care is changing and becoming more "health care" as shown by the increase in home care, patient centered medical homes, and independent living retirement communities.

Perhaps the greatest need in terms of numbers of clients continues to be in the areas of health and wellness. Health and wellness concerns are becoming more universal and RDNs must take the leadership role especially since the fundamentals of food and nutrition impact every aspect of health and wellness. The general public is becoming more aware of the relationship between nutrition and healthy lifestyles (including mental health). The Internet provides much information that has yet to be confirmed and needs translation and verification by dietetic professionals.

The potential for an exciting specific area of practice is nutritional genomics for which RDNs will be key personnel and need education and skills not currently being attained by enough practitioners or students to fill the need.[15] Nutrigenomics provides the potential for food and dietary intake modifications in preventing disease, individualizing (personalized nutrition) treatment of disease, and in health and wellness. Ongoing research in this area illustrated the need for knowledge in nutrition, genomics, bioinformatics, molecular biology, and epidemiology. Dietitians in research are and will continue to be engaged in determining new high tech methods of dietary assessment, futuristic food preparation, and working with food scientists to understand the complexities of food composition in nano- and micronutrient bases. This emerging area requires a full understanding, interpretation, and communication of complex genetic testing results to assess disease risk.[16]

In the present healthcare climate, there are increasing opportunities for the RDN to advocate for inclusion and to demonstrate value and willingness to collaborate for new partnerships. Examples are in patient-centered medical homes and accountability care organizations.[17] This new area is structured to reward improved outcomes of programs and treatments and since dietitians are attuned to wellness and disease prevention, they are well placed to take advantage of these opportunities.

A career model described as a "lattice career ladder" allows persons to define their careers in ways that are flexible and that fulfill gaps in services.[18] As priorities and circumstances change, careers may be customized for the best and most supportive environment.

COMMUNICATIONS AND TECHNOLOGY

Trends in communications, informatics, and technology change and progress on a regular basis. Business, industry, and retail establishments provide programs, products, and services for the public and it is up to the consumer to discern among these what is reliable and in their best interests.

A few dietitians have been employed with food and nutrition product companies for years. There is a need and great opportunities for dietitians to provide leadership with corporations and businesses in ways that help the public obtain accurate and useful nutrition information.

Communications remain the life blood of professionals, organizations, and business entities. Traditional means of communication such as face to face meetings and written communication are increasingly replaced by teleconferencing, webinars, emails, and other social media means. And the media technology itself keeps changing and evolving. As future practice options open, there will be an even greater need to recognize the many communication modes available to reach consumers and for dietitians to continually update their own professional expertise. This is also true in the area of personalized nutrition counseling and nutrition education (especially games for children, teens, and possibly other age groups).

Telenutrition is increasingly offered today by telephone consultation through dietitian call centers and by other website tools for dietary assessment, social networking video-based application, smartphone texting, and others. The entry-level RD will need to keep abreast of the new technologies and their professional, personal, legal, and ethical responsibilities in providing telenutrition. These responsibilities include digital computers regulatory requirements and privacy laws among others.[19]

Mobile APPS are discussed by Stein[20] as an advanced way for reaching clients for remote counseling. This has the potential of reaching many consumers and clients outside the traditional office environment. There are legal and policy considerations, as with any technological communication means, but this is a widespread trend that health professionals need to be knowledgeable about for application to their practice. Another opportunity for future RDNs to be assertive is partnering with professionals in information technology, engineers, and those inventing games and other hand held devices to ensure accurate food and nutrition is included in their products.

FOOD AND THE FOOD SUPPLY

Food, food safety, food sustainability, food labeling, and genetically modified foods are all topics of consumer interest and concern. At the same time, the U.S. food supply does not match up well with dietary advice and food policy. For instance, the Healthy Eating Index-2010 pinpoints fruit, vegetables, whole grains, dairy, and sodium at less than sufficient availability.[21,22] From a public health perspective, this can be problematic in regard to access and intake of the right kind of food. Health problems, it should be noted, also arise from poor food choices as well as from poverty, lack of reliable information, or lack of access to grocery stores and other sources of food.

A framework for food and water systems that ensures equitable and optimal access now and in the future was developed by the Hunger and Environmental Nutrition Practice Group.[23] Several principles are incorporated[24]:

- Nutrition and health from safe and secure food and water supplies.
- Social, cultural, and ethical capital that promotes cultural diversity; empowers social responsibility and community engagement; advances ethical, humane, and fair treatment of individuals and animals.
- Environmental stewardship that conserves, protects, and renews natural resources.
- Economic vitality to build community wealth and viable economics.

The involvement of RDNs and DTRs in dispersing information about food and the food supply toward improving the health of Americans will be even more critical in the future. Consumer attitudes and beliefs about food are often shaped by the media and through advertising. The Dietary Guidelines for Americans and MyPlate form the foundation for good food choices and should be strongly promoted by all healthcare groups.

Dietitians providing input into policy formation, such as the national Farm Bill, the dietary guidelines, and other governmental policies about food and nutrition is a way of influencing food availability and other issues regarding food and the food supply.[25] Some of the current issues receiving attention are more emphasis on fresh, local, and organic foods and more federal funding for fruits and vegetable production. In the latest version of the Farm Bill, funds were also provided to help farmers transition from conventional to organic farming. Still controversial are subsidies for dairy producers and corn growers. RDNs should be involved in public debates over any of these issues that could preclude an adequate food supply for all Americans.

Legislation and regulations have a direct impact on dietetic practice through actions affecting health care, food, and consumer issues. The Dietary

Guidelines for Americans, with an emphasis on prevention of chronic disease through food choices, continue to be controversial. Surveys have shown that they are not universally followed and that the agricultural system is not fully compatible with the guidelines. This presents an urgency for dietitians to take the lead in educating other professionals, individuals, and the public about best food practices for health and wellness and to document their preeminence of knowledge and skills in this area. A relatively untapped area of application of the Dietary Guidelines is beginning to emerge. A recent report in Food Management magazine documents the implementation of the Centers for Disease Control and Prevention (CDC) "healthy workplace foodservice guidelines" as an example of consumers demanding healthier food choices for an active lifestyle.[26]

Food safety is an ongoing concern for all dietitians given the regular media reports of outbreaks due to food handling and contamination. Community dietitians and nutritionists have many opportunities for raising awareness of safety risks and ways to prevent illness through good practices. Through programs such as Child School Nutrition, the Elderly Nutrition Program, WIC, and the Supplemental Nutrition Assistance Program (SNAP), consumers can be reached directly with food safety information critical to health. Oversight of regulations and enforcement of sanitation codes and safety measures in effect are also important steps in safeguarding health. Most of these food safety issues provide an opportunity for partnering of RDNs and microbiologists, chefs, sanitarian specialists, and other professionals.

MANAGEMENT AND LEADERSHIP

Although only about 12 percent of RDNs identify their area of practice as Food and Nutrition Management, all dietitians are managers in certain ways. An emphasis on managerial competence is needed more than ever as opportunities for expanded interprofessional employment occur. The food and foodservice environment will drive changes in the profession and the role of food service and the manager will become more important at the same time. The ability to manage budgets, personnel production, and service is a complex and challenging undertaking. Managerial skills acquired through both education and experience help prepare individuals to assume positions of increasing responsibility and, in turn, better salaries.

Management skills have been identified as a weakness among entry-level RDNs by employers.[27] The Academy has identified management competencies in food and nutrition services in health care but it has been suggested that educational competencies need to be reexamined to promote management as an essential part of the dietetics curriculum and professional practice. Management is a critical skill in all areas of practice. Employers emphasize the need for RDNs who can see the big picture and think strategically, run and justify programs, understand health care as a business, add value, and are entrepreneurial.[27]

Hospitals are challenged to offer healthier food in all areas; school nutrition program directors are required to respond to new regulations, public eating places are increasingly required to make nutrition information available and some policy makers are dealing with public initiatives that promote healthier practices through taxes or other directives. The challenges are very real and management expertise in all areas of practice is needed to help meet the needs in food service and in programs for the public.

Productivity and accountability are integral parts of a manager's responsibility. Managers are expected to make decisions in the best interests of the system—not just a department. Critical, forward-looking thinking is valued and is an essential part of ensuring productivity of a unit. In this regard, another dimension—that of "polarity thinking" is necessarily a part of what a manager must do. Polarities are defined as interdependent yet potentially polar opposite pairs of values.[28] An example is a manager or an institution holding to the highest quality of food service but at the lowest cost. Another example is a school that wants to promote good eating for students but also provides vending machines with junk food for income. A community dietitian may be faced with advising clients to follow the Dietary Guidelines when they lack access to good sources of fruits and vegetables or they lack knowledge or can't afford them. Polarity thinking requires skill in balancing both ends of such situations within the context of the organization. Even though they may be competing values, they must be managed effectively, and simultaneously.

Leadership skills for the dietitian are essential in communications, in demonstrating ability and professionalism, and in building brands and businesses. Consultants in all areas of practice must display leadership skill in order to be successful. Leadership involves keeping abreast of future and emerging trends, networking and sharing knowledge, being innovative and creative, and even risk-taking.

SUMMARY

The future offers many challenges and opportunities for dietitians. Food and nutrition are gaining prime importance in the issues of health and wellness at no time in the past as there been so much interest in nutrition and food science. Dietetic professionals must "seize the moment" as suggested by Healy and be ready to embrace the changes and challenges of the future. Educational standards will change as practice requirements evolve and educators respond to change in the best interests of their students. The workplace increasingly offers new and innovative areas for practice especially for the professional who is willing to take the risk for a new and exciting career. Some things will not change. Continuing education with increased knowledge and expertise will always be needed in keeping with communication and technological changes. Effective managers and leaders in food service systems and nutrition systems as well as in all other areas of practice will continue to be valued and valuable to patients, client, student, customers, and the public.

DEFINITIONS

Healthy Eating Index. A measure of diet quality that assesses conformity to recommended dietary intake.
Food sustainability. Describes adequacy of the food supply.
Paradigm. A model or template for how things should be done.
Polarity. Pertaining to the opposite ends or sides of an object or subject.
Productivity. The output efficiency of something produced or measured.
Standards. Statements of specifications by which something may be tested or measured.

REFERENCES

1. Healy, B. Why Nutrition and Genomics Are Important. "The Promise of Nutrigenomics." Institute of Medicine. *Nutrigenomics and Beyond: Informing the Future—Workshop Summary.* (Washington, DC: The National Academies Press, 2007).
2. Kicklighter, J.R., M.M. Cluskey, A.M. Hunter, N.K. Nyland, and B.A. Spear. "Council on Future Practice Visioning Report and Consensus Agreement for Moving Toward the Continuum of Dietetics Education, Credentialing, and Practice." *J Acad Nutr Diet* 113, no. 12 (2013): 1710–1731.

3. Connor, S.L. "Our Academy's First Hundred Years—and the Next." *J Acad Nutr Diet* 115, no. 2 (2015): 179.
4. Institute of Medicine. "The IOM's Future Practice Educational Recommendations." 2012.
5. Rationale for Future Education Preparation of Nutrition and Dietetics Practitioners. 2015. www.eatright.org/ACEND
6. Eliot, K.A. "The Value in Interprofesssional Collaborative-Ready Nutrition and Dietetics Practitioners." *J Acad Nutr Diet* 115, no. 10 (2015): 1578–1588.
7. See Note 4.
8. Department of Nutritional Sciences. Oklahoma State University. 2015–2016. (With permission.)
9. See Note 2.
10. Federal Register. Medicare and Medicaid Programs; regulatory provisions to promote program efficiency, transparency and burden reduction. www.federalregister.gov. May 12, 2014. (4/4/16).
11. Martin, A.L., and R.D. Lipman. "The Future of Diabetes Education: Expanded Opportunities and Roles for Diabetes Educators." *Diabetes Educ* 39, no. 4 (2013): 436–446.
12. See Note 11.
13. Sauer, H. "Results of the 2013 Non-RD Baccalaureate DPD Graduate Dietetics Practice Audit." *J Acad Nutr Diet* 114, no. 10 (2014): 1630–1639.
14. Smart, H. "Nutrition Students Gain Skills from Motivational Interviewing Curriculum." *J Acad Nutr Diet* 114, no. 11 (2014): 1712–1717.
15. See Note 1.
16. www.eatright.org/ACEND Standards.
17. Boyce, B. "Emerging Paradigms in Dietetics Practice and Health Care: Patient-Centered Medical Homes and Accountable Organizations." *J Acad Nutr Diet* 115, no. 11 (2015): 1765–1770.
18. Gilbride, J.A., S.C. Parks, and R. Dowling. "The Potential of Nutrition and Dietetics Practice." *Topics in Clinical Nutrition* 28, no. 3 (2013): 220–232.
19. Benko, C., and S. Vickberg. "The Corporate Lattice: A Strategic Response to the Changing World of Work." *Deloitte Review* 8 (2011): 95–97.
20. Stein, K. "Remote Nutrition Counseling: Considerations in a New Channel for Client Communications." *J Acad Nutr Diet* 115, no. 10 (2015): 1561–1576.
21. Miller, P.E., J. Reedy, S.I. Kirkpatrick, S. Krebs-Smith. "The United States Food Supply Is not Consistent with Dietary Guidance: Evidence from an Evaluation Using the Healthy Eating Index-2010." *J Acad Nutr Diet* 115, no. 1 (2015): 95–100.
22. Zizza, C.A. "Policies and Politics of the US Food Supply." *J Acad Nutr Diet* 115, no. 1 (2015): 27–30.
23. Tagtow, A., K. Robien, R. Bergquist, M. Bruening, L. Dierks, B.E. Hartman, R. Robinson-O'Brien, et al. "Academy of Nutrition and Dietetics: Standards of Professional Performance for Registered Dietitian Nutritionists (Competent, Proficient, and Expert) in Sustainable, Resilient, and healthy Food and Water Systems." *J Acad Nutr Diet* 114, no. 3 (2014): 475–488.

24. See Note 23.

25. Taylor, M. "CDC Builds New Café on Healthy-Eating Guidelines." *Food Management* 10, no. 2 (2016): 19.

26. Berthelson, R.M., W.C. Barkley, P.M. Oliver, V. McLymont, R. Puckett. "Academy of Nutrition and Dietetics: Revised 2014 Standards of Professional Performance for Registered Dietitian Nutritionists in Management of Food and Nutrition Systems." *J Acad Nutr Diet* 114, no. 7 (2014): 1104–1112.

27. "Practice Paper of the Academy of Nutrition and Dietetics: Principles of Productivity in Food and Nutrition Services: Applications in the 21st Century Health Care Reform Era." *J Acad Nutr Diet* 115, no. 7 (2015): 1141–1147.

28. Cluskey, M., B. Gerald, and M. Gregoire. "Management in Dietetics: Are We Prepared for the Future?" *J Acad Nutr Diet* 112, Suppl. 2 (2012): S34–S35.

Code of Ethics for the Profession of Dietetics and Process for Consideration of Ethics Issues (2009)

PREAMBLE

The American Dietetic Association (ADA) and its credentialing agency, the Commission on Dietetic Registration (CDR), believe it is in the best interest of the profession and the public it serves to have a Code of Ethics in place that provides guidance to dietetic practitioners in their professional practice and conduct. Dietetics practitioners have voluntarily adopted this Code of Ethics to reflect the values and ethical principles guiding the dietetics profession and to set forth commitments and obligations of the dietetics practitioner to the public, clients, the profession, colleagues, and other professionals. The current Code of Ethics was approved on June 2, 2009, by the ADA Board of Directors, House of Delegates, and the Commission on Dietetic Registration.

APPLICATION

The Code of Ethics applies to the following practitioners:

   (a) In its entirety to members of ADA who are Registered Dietitians or Dietetic Technicians.

   (b) Except for sections dealing solely with the credential, to all members of ADA who are not RDs or DTRs.

   (c) Except for aspects dealing solely with membership, to all RDs and DTRs who are not members of ADA.

FUNDAMENTAL PRINCIPLES

1. The dietetics practitioner conducts himself/herself with honesty, integrity, and fairness.

2. The dietetics practitioner supports and promotes high standards of professional practice. The dietetics practitioner accepts the obligation to protect clients, the public, and the profession by upholding the Code of Ethics for the profession of dietetics and by reporting perceived violations of the Code through the processes established by ADA and its credentialing agency, CDR.

3. The dietetics practitioner considers the health, safety, and welfare of the public at all times.

4. The dietetics practitioner complies with all laws and regulations applicable or related to the profession or to the practitioner's ethical obligations as described in this Code.

5. The dietetics practitioner provides professional services with objectivity and with respect for the unique needs and values of individuals.

6. The dietetics practitioner does not engage in false or misleading practices or communications.

7. The dietetics practitioner withdraws from professional practice when unable to fulfill his or her professional duties and responsibilities to clients and others.

8. The dietetics practitioner recognizes and exercises professional judgment within the limits of his or her qualifications and collaborates with others, seeks counsel, or makes referrals as appropriate.

9. The dietetics practitioner treats clients and patients with respect and consideration.
10. The dietetics practitioner protects confidential information and makes full disclosure about any limitations on his or her ability to guarantee full confidentiality.
11. The dietetics practitioner, in dealing with and providing services to clients and others, complies with the same principles set forth above.
12. The dietetics practitioner practices dietetics based on evidence-based principles and current information.
13. The dietetics practitioner presents reliable and substantiated information and interprets controversial information without personal bias, recognizing that legitimate differences of opinion exist.
14. The dietetics practitioner assumes a life-long responsibility and accountability for personal competence in practice, consistent with accepted professional standards, continually striving to increase professional knowledge and skills and to apply them in practice.
15. The dietetics practitioner is alert to the occurrence of a real or potential conflict of interest and takes appropriate action whenever a conflict arises.
16. The dietetics practitioner permits the use of his or her name for the purpose of certifying that dietetics services have been rendered only if he or she has provided or supervised the provision of those services.
17. The dietetics practitioner accurately presents professional qualifications and credentials.
18. The dietetics practitioner does not invite, accept, or offer gifts, monetary incentives, or other considerations that affect or reasonably give an appearance of affecting his or her professional judgment.
19. The dietetics practitioner demonstrates respect for the values, rights, knowledge, and skills of colleagues and other professionals.

Adapted from *Journal of the American Dietetic Association*, 109(8) "The American Dietetic Association/Commission on Dietetic Registration Code of Ethics for the Profession of Dietetics and Process for Consideration of Ethics Issues," pp. 1461–1467, Copyright © 2009, with permission from Elsevier.

Dietetics Career Development Guide

Dietetics Career Development Guide

Expert
Builds and maintains knowledge, skills and credentials

Advanced Practice
Continues at the highest level of knowledge, skills & behaviors including leadership, vision and/or advanced credential

Proficient
Operational Skills Obtained and Adeptly Practiced Long Term
May Begin to Acquire Specialist Credentials

Competent
Start of Practice after Registration
(Generally, the First Three Years of Practice)

Standards of Practice (SOP)

Standards of Professional Performance (SOPP)

Beginner (Learning Phase)

| CP (Coordinated Program) | Supervised Practice DI (Dietetic Internship) | DTP (Dietetic Technician Program) |

Novice

| CP (Coordinated Program) | Didactic Education DPD (Didactic Program in Dietetics) | DTP (Dietetic Technician Program) |

RD Pathways   **DTR Pathway**

Focus Area   Knowledge & Skills

Life-long Learning and Professional Development ...

EDUCATION FOR ENTRY INTO CAREER
Associate, Baccalaureate or Advanced Degree

Definition of Dietetics: Dietetics is the integration, application and communication of principles derived from food, nutrition, social, business and basic sciences, to achieve and maintain optimal nutrition status of individuals through the development, provision and management of effective food and nutrition services in a variety of settings.

© Academy of Nutrition and Dietetics. Reprinted by permission of Academy of Nutrition and Dietetics.

Glossary

Academy of Nutrition and Dietetics. The professional organization for dietitians. Formerly known as the *American Dietetic Association.*

Accreditation. The process whereby a private nongovernmental agency or association grants public recognition to an institution or an individual who meets necessary qualifications and periodic evaluation.

Advanced practice. Effective discharge of job requirements that demonstrates a high level of skills, knowledge, and behaviors.

Advanced study. Study beyond the traditional baccalaureate level.

Anorexia nervosa. An eating disorder characterized by a preoccupation with dieting and thinness that leads to excessive weight loss.

Assessment. The process of evaluating actions or conditions to base additional activity.

Benchmarking. Comparing performance measures for the development of better methods and procedures.

Bulimia nervosa. An eating disorder involving frequent episodes of binge eating followed by purging, also leading to excessive weight loss.

Bylaws. Authoritative rules governing an association or group.

Cardiovascular nutrition. Application of medical nutrition therapy for those with heart and blood vessel conditions or to prevent the diseases.

Certification. The process by which a nongovernmental agency or association grants recognition to an individual who has met certain predetermined qualifications specified by that agency or association (e.g., registration for dietitians and dietetic technicians administered by the CDR).

Chief executive officer (CEO). A person employed by the association to direct the headquarters office operations and implement the programs and fiscal affairs of the association. May also serve as an official spokesperson for the Academy on direction of the board of directors.

Client. The recipient of services or products.

Clinical dietetics. The area of practice in which persons with illness or injury involving nutritional factors are treated using assessment, planning, and implementing nutrition care plans.

Clinical nutrition services. Activities provided in the practice of clinical dietetics, such as medical nutrition therapy and counseling.

Coach. A person who guides, inspires, and motivates.

Cognitive skills. The application of intellectual capabilities to accomplish objectives.

Community health. Health measures applied to groups of people.

Community nutrition. Nutrition issues and services provided for groups of people.

Consultant. A skilled and knowledgeable person qualified to give expert professional advice.

Coordinated program (CP). A degree undergraduate program that combines didactic and experiential learning.

Credentialing. Formal recognition of professional or technical competence as by certification or licensure.

Diet therapy. Treatment by diet; a term now replaced by *clinical nutrition therapy* or *medical nutrition therapy* .

Dietetic practice group (DPG). An organized group of Academy of Nutrition and Dietetics members with similar interests in an area of practice or a particular subject area.

Dietetic technician. A graduate of an approved dietetic technician program.

Dietitian. A professional who translates the science of food and nutrition to enhance the health and well-being of individuals and groups.

Disordered eating. Abnormal eating patterns.

Diversity. A term with multiple, subjective definitions; may refer to age, physical ability, religion, socioeconomic status, sex, race, ethnicity, or other factors.

Education. The systematic instruction and training designed to impart knowledge and develop a skill.

Entrepreneur. An innovative person who initiates a new activity, career, or business.

Evidence-based research. The compilation of research studies that, together, allows for a decision regarding application to practice.

Evidence-based. Action based on research data and evaluation of outcomes.

Extended care facility. An institution that extends health care beyond the acute care setting when long-term term care is needed.

Food Assistance. Food that is provided in feeding programs or by voucher to buy food.

Food production. The process of preparing and serving food, including purchasing, storage, and processing.

Food service systems. Activities that together form the inputs, transformation, and outputs that make up an entire food operation.

Food services. Production and service of food; also refers to the unit or group responsible for feeding groups.

Food sustainability. Describes adequacy of the food supply.

Governance. Activities involved in conducting the affairs of an organization.

Health promotion. Education and preventive measures directed toward healthy populations to foster wellness and prevention of disease.

Healthy Eating Index. A measure of diet quality that assesses conformity to recommended dietary intake.

Human resources. The personnel in an organization.

Instruction. The activity by which knowledge or teaching is imparted.

Intrapraneur. A person within an organization who develops new ideas or services.

Leadership. The qualities that allow an individual to influence the actions of others.

Licensure. Process by which a government agency grants permission to an individual to engage in a given occupation upon finding that the applicant has attained the minimal degree of competency necessary to ensure that the public health, safety, and welfare are reasonably well protected.

Long-term care. Assistance provided over time to people with chronic health conditions and/or physical disabilities and those who are unable to care for themselves.

Managed care. A system of care administered by an entity outside a hospital or healthcare institution in which access, cost, and quality of care are controlled by direct intervention before or during service for purposes of creating efficiencies and/or reducing costs.

Management. The administration and coordination of the activities and functions in an organizational unit.

Medical nutrition therapy. The application of nutrition in the management of illness or injury.

Mentor. A person who teaches and guides by instructing, demonstrating, encouraging, and role modeling.

Networking. Activities directed toward making connections with others through varied contacts.

Nutrition assessment. Evaluation of an individual's nutritional status based on anthropometric, biochemical, clinical, and dietary information.

Nutritionist. A professional with academic credentials in nutrition; he or she may also be an RD.

Outcomes research. Studies that focus on results of interventions and application of research results.

Outpatient clinic. Treatment area of a hospital or healthcare facility in which patients are treated on an outpatient basis.

Paradigm. A model or template for how things should be done.

Polarity. Pertaining to the opposite ends or sides of an object or subject.

Political Action Committee. Group pooling of money to support political candidates or office holders.

Practitioner. One who practices in a profession or occupation.

Preceptor. A person who guides, mentors, and evaluates a student during supervised practice.

Private practice. Self-employment in which a person manages his or her own working career.

Productivity. The output efficiency of something produced or measured.

Program planning. Needs assessment and action plans to meet needs.

Psychomotor skills. The ability to perform physical tasks based on knowing or thinking.

Public Policy. The promotion of a law, a regulation, or a recommendation targeted to the public at large.

Quality assurance. The certification of the continual, optimal, effective, and efficient outcomes of a service or program.

Quality improvement. The provision of service that assures the needs of those served are met through adherence to high standards of care.

Registered dietitian (RD). A dietitian who has fulfilled the eligibility requirements of the Commission on Dietetic Registration.

Registration. See Certification.

Regulation. Written rules to activate laws passed through legislation.

Research. Systematic investigation leading to new knowledge or new applications of known information. To conduct research, a question is formulated, a literature search is conducted, experimental activities are applied, and results are recorded.

Resource allocation. The equitable distribution of financial, physical, and human capital.

Resource management. The handling of money, equipment and supplies, or personnel essential to the administration of an organizational unit.

Scope of practice. Extent of or dimensions of activities performed in an area of practice.

Specialist. One who possesses a proficient level of knowledge, skill, and experience to qualify for a specific credential.

Sports nutrition. The area of nutrition specific to the needs of those who participate in sports activities.

Standard. A measure of proficiency at an established level.

Standards. Statements of specifications by which something may be tested or measured.

Strategic plan. Plans and strategies that shape the overall activities and functions of an organization.

Strategic planning. Long-range planning that involves data gathering, data analysis, development of goals and objectives, and action plans.

Supervised practice. Learning experiences associated with activities guided by a leader or preceptor.

Surveillance. Research-based activities to assess a program's reach and impact.

Training. Actions by which persons are brought to a desired standard of efficiency or behavior by instruction and practice.

Wellness. State of optimal health and the absence of disease.

Index

Page numbers followed by *f* or *t* represent figures and tables.

Dietary reference intakes (DRIs), 134
Dietetic assistant, 102
Dietetic practice doctorate degree, 43
Dietetic practice groups (DPGs), 12
  defined, 17
  descriptions and purpose of, 28–31,
    29–31*t*
  dues for, 24
  networking through, 28
  subunits of, 28
Dietetics. *See also* Clinical dietetics
  educational preparation for.
    See Education
  employment survey for, 11–12, 12*t*
  history of, 1–17. *See also* History of
    dietetics
  as profession, 8–9
  standards of practice, 148
Dietetics Career Development Guide, 59
Dietetics Practice-Based Research Network
    (DPBRN), 214, 217
Dietetics technician, registered
    (DTRs), 230
  practice of dietetics, 233
  role in dispersing information, 236
Dietetic technician (DT) program, 39, 40
Dietetic technicians, registered (DTRs),
    125, 130, 142
  career development for, 57
  credentialing of, 58–60
  defined, 17
  educational requirements. *See* Education
  employment settings of, 57–58, 93–94,
    93–94*t*. *See also* Employment
  employment survey for, 11–12, 12*t*
  legal regulation statutes for, 66–67
  management activities of, 109–110,
    109–110*t*
  recertification of, 64–65
  registration eligibility pathway for, 58–60
  responsibilities of, 102
  salaries of, 31–33, 32*t*
  scope of practice for, 75
Dietitians
  in business and communications,
    158–161
  in cardiovascular nutrition, 165–166
  for clinical dietetics. *See* Clinical dietetics

as consultants, 143–154. *See also*
    Consultants
  defined, 17, 52, 92
  educational activities of, 193, 193*t*
  education for. *See* Education
  educator role of, 192–193, 198–205
  employment settings of, 93–94, 93–94*t*
  employment survey for, 11–12, 12*t*
  ethics and, 77–78
  expanded opportunities for, 117
  expanded roles, 117–118
  in health and wellness programs, 161–169
  legal considerations for, 84–85
  means of communicating nutrition,
    205, 205*f*
  as mentor, 160
  networking, 160–161
  nontraditional choice of career for,
    158–161
  in private practice, 159
  professional practice of. *See* Professional
    practice
  salaries of, 31–33, 32*t*
  in sports nutrition, 162–165
  strategic skill building, 161
  teaching skills, 194–195
  in treatment of disordered eating,
    168–169
  in wellness and health promotion,
    166–168
Dietitians in Business and Communications
    practice group, 169
Dietitians of Canada, 163
Dietotherapy, 5
Diet therapy, 2–4, 92, 105
Disease prevention, 124–125
Disordered eating, 168–169
Distance education, 46–47
District and state associations, 33
Diversity, 23, 80, 88
Doctoral degree, 43
DPD. *See* Didactic program in dietetics
    (DPD)
Dreyfus model of skill acquisition, 59
Drucker, Peter, 175
Dues/maintenance fees
  for academy membership, 5, 24, 27
  for dietetic practice groups, 28